CURRICULUM-BASED MEASUREMENT
Assessing Special Children

The Guilford School Practitioner Series

EDITORS
STEPHEN N. ELLIOTT, Ph.D.
University of Wisconsin—Madison
JOSEPH C. WITT, Ph.D.
Louisiana State University, Baton Rouge

Academic Skills Problems: Direct Assessment and Intervention
EDWARD S. SHAPIRO

Curriculum-Based Measurement: Assessing Special Children
MARK R. SHINN (ED.)

Suicide Intervention in the Schools
SCOTT POLAND

Problems in Written Expression: Assessment and Remediation
SHARON BRADLEY-JOHNSON AND JUDI F. LESIAK

CURRICULUM-BASED MEASUREMENT
Assessing Special Children

Edited by
MARK R. SHINN, Ph.D.
University of Oregon

THE GUILFORD PRESS
New York   London

© 1989 The Guilford Press
A Division of Guilford Publications, Inc.
72 Spring Street, New York, NY 10012

Printed in the United States of America

Last digit is print number: 9   8   7   6   5   4   3   2   1

Library of Congress Cataloging-in-Publication Data
Curriculum-based measurement: assessing special children/
    edited by Mark R. Shinn.
        p.   cm. — (The Guilford school practitioner series)
    Bibliography: p.
    Includes index.
    1. Curriculum-based assessment—United States.   2. Educational
tests and measurements—United States.   3. Special education—United
States.   I. Shinn, Mark R.   II. Series.
LB3060.32.C74C87 1989
371.9'0973—dc19
ISBN 0–89862–352–9   88–24599
ISBN 0–89862–231–X (pbk.)   CIP

Preface and Acknowledgments

This book is the second major product of a group of educators' efforts to apply behaviorally based methodologies to the evaluation and improvement of special education students' instructional programs. The first, *Data Based Program Modification (DBPM)*, by Stanley L. Deno and Phyllis K. Mirkin, was published by the Council of Exceptional Children in 1977. That book culminated more than 5 years of training special education resource teachers at Seward School in the Minneapolis Public Schools. Its goals focused on the use of behaviorally based strategies and single-case study designs to get teachers to evaluate what worked with individual students.

This volume represents the outcome of 10 more years of work in both university and field-based settings. In contrast to the *DBPM* text, which served as the precursor to curriculum-based measurement (CBM), this book is based on a more integrated and empirically supported foundation. Additionally, the initial work on decision making regarding the effectiveness of individual students' instructional programs has been expanded to represent a system for making a continuum of special education decisions. Support for the underlying research foundation for CBM has come primarily from the United States Department of Education, Special Education Programs, from a variety of funding programs. Other sources of the data base include the local efforts of school psychologists and special educators in public schools.

The book is organized into two major parts. In the first part, a general background in CBM is provided. If the history of other educational measurement systems or procedures runs true, curriculum-based measurement is susceptible to the risk of assuming the appearance of a technology. That is, the measurement system that is used to make a set of related special education decisions may be translated into an atheoretical set of testing procedures. In fact, CBM is more than a measurement system. It provides the foundation for implementation of a problem-solving approach to the instructional problems of students. In Chapter 1, Deno sets the occasion for understanding CBM as it relates to definitions of special education and the children that it serves. He establishes the underlying philosophical background of CBM, its tenets, and the assumptions that make it more than a set of simple "tests."

In Chapter 2, Marston presents the basic background information on what CBM is. As part of his chapter, Marston provides a rationale for CBM as an alternative assessment and decision-making system, reviewing current assessment practices in a framework of both psychometric properties and social policy. His chapter also details the basic elements of the essential features of CBM, distinguishing it from other curriculum-based models.

An example of how the features of CBM described by Marston are operationalized is presented in Chapter 3. This chapter takes a case-study approach with a fourth-grade student to show how CBM is used as part of the special education decision-making process, from the point of special education referral to the periodic and annual review process.

The second part of this book focuses on procedures for implementation of CBM in school settings. The chapters are sequenced via a set of typical consecutive decisions that are made with students considered handicapped by school systems. In Chapter 4, CBM procedures for making special education screening and eligibility decisions are detailed. The chapter incorporates the development and use of local norms at various levels (e.g., classrooms, school districts) to assist in the decision-making process.

The primary value of CBM is its use in evaluating student instructional outcomes. CBM has contributed uniquely to this process in two ways: (1) explicit observable individual education plan (IEP) objectives that can be measured routinely, and (2) standardized and frequent data collection and interpretation strategies for determining success. The former are presented in Chapter 5. Fuchs and I specify the procedures and factors to consider when writing data-based goals for IEPs. A rationale for explicit and measurable goals is provided, and specific methods for selecting IEP goal materials and criterion for success are elucidated. The latter, standardized, frequent data collection and interpretation strategies for monitoring progress, are explored by Fuchs in

Chapter 6. Using the area of reading as a prototype for the basic skill areas, she delineates the essential tasks that must be accomplished to evaluate an initial teaching program's success.

Periodic review, annual review, and exit decisions also are important ones for evaluating student outcomes. School psychologists typically do not participate in them; further, the basis of these decisions usually lies in data that are either subjective or technically inadequate. In Chapter 7, Allen contributes further to the continuity of special education decision making by describing the use of CBM to make these decisions. Methods for making normative and individually referenced decisions are presented.

Finally, CBM data collected for making all of the special education decisions for individual students can constitute the basic datum for evaluating the programs provided to groups of students. In Chapter 8, Tindal covers three methods of aggregating CBM data across students, norm-referenced, criterion-referenced, and individually referenced, that allow for conclusions of effect to be drawn.

This book is the product of the efforts of many persons, in both university and public school settings. It represents the collective efforts of the authors and others to provide a data-based special education decision-making framework—it is the written product of a group of people (Allen, Fuchs, Marston, Tindal, and I, as well as Caren Wesson, whom circumstance precluded from formal participation in this work) who happened to coalesce at the University of Minnesota in the 1970s and worked with Stanley L. Deno. Primary acknowledgment for this book must go to him. It is Stan Deno who has seriously influenced all of our professional (and personal) lives. For those of us who are school psychologists, Stan provided us with a viable alternative to the traditional training we received and the practices we observed. His influence on our work and lives has been immeasurable.

We also wish to acknowledge the contribution of the late Phyllis K. Mirkin. Phyllis began her work in CBM in the early 1970s as a doctoral student in Stan's initial work on data-based program modification. Subsequently, Phyllis became Stan's colleague in the seminal research efforts in CBM as Associate Director of the Institute for Research on Learning Disabilities at Minnesota. Her tireless efforts at managing the CBM research, writing, and the "unruly bunch" that served as research assistants are substantive.

One of my favorite "Deno-isms" is that "university professors are trained to admire problems, not solve them!" Thus, it is most important to acknowledge the efforts of the field-based practitioners who have attempted to use CBM to provide a different approach to special education service delivery. Gary Germann, Director of Special Education in the Pine County Special Education Cooperative, took the pioneering steps to fully operationalize CBM into an integrated decision-making system. His Cooperative served as the primary site for initial research on implementation. Gary's efforts and ideas, most often carried out with great success, provided the foundation for solid school-based practices that enabled other districts to implement CBM successfully. It is likely that without his work, implementation of CBM would have remained in the "ivory tower."

Acknowledgments also must be given to the leadership of Drs. Deanne Magnusson, Keith Kromer, and Judith Brown in implementing of CBM in the Minneapolis Public Schools. Their commitment to a data-based decision-making process and concomitant improvement in interventions for handicapped and nonhandicapped students provided (and continues to provide) an environment conducive to CBM. Their teachers and classrooms have been involved in continuing efforts at innovative CBM practices, procedures, and federally supported cooperative research with the University of Minnesota. Like Gary Germann, they have participated in innumerable meetings to argue for "changing the system" that, in its short lifespan, has become calcified.

It is unfortunate that space does not permit acknowledging individually all the other administrators and the special and regular education teachers who have implemented this program. CBM has facilitated the linking up of practicing school psychologists with teachers and the teaching process. I am a better school psychologist for the teaching I received from my school colleagues, Lionel Blatchley, Carol Rye, Heather Sillers, Vivian Lytle, Meredith LaGuarde, Karen Erickson, Linda Locher, and Margarita Aguilera-Tookey among others.

Stephen Elliott and Joseph Witt provided valuable support during the preparation of this text, including timely prompts to meet deadlines, patient understanding when some deadlines had to be modified, and their timely yet high-quality editing.

Finally, but most especially, I want to thank my wife, Judy, and my son, Peter, for their patience, understanding, support, and encouragement during this project.

Mark R. Shinn

Contents

Contributors

DONALD ALLEN, Ph.D., K–12 Special Education Programs, Minneapolis Public Schools, Minneapolis, MN.

STANLEY L. DENO, Ph.D., Department of Educational Psychology, University of Minnesota, Minneapolis, MN.

LYNN S. FUCHS, Ph.D., Peabody College, Vanderbilt University, Nashville, TN.

DOUGLAS B. MARSTON, Ph.D., Department of Special Education, Minneapolis Public Schools, Minneapolis, MN.

MARK R. SHINN, Ph.D., University of Oregon, Eugene, OR.

GERALD A. TINDAL, Ph.D., University of Oregon, Eugene, OR.

1

Curriculum-Based Measurement and Special Education Services: A Fundamental and Direct Relationship

Stanley L. Deno

Curriculum-based measurement (CBM) is a systematic set of procedures that produces a data base for making special education decisions. Evidence has accumulated not only that using the curriculum as a basis for measurement is feasible but also that appropriate use of CBM results in more effective instructional interventions for students with mild handicaps. Although the effectiveness of CBM as an instrument for improving student achievement must be the first consideration for professionals interested in adopting CBM approaches, an understanding of the assumptions underlying the use of CBM in providing services to mildly handicapped students is also important. Knowledge of those assumptions provides a basis for understanding the approach taken to providing services in school systems that have adopted curriculum-based data as a basis for special education decision making.

SPECIAL EDUCATION AS PROBLEM SOLVING

Special education is often referred to as a service delivery system (Deno, 1970). Such a characterization is useful, especially from an administrative perspective, but it also has the effect of focusing attention primarily on administrative arrangements (i.e., on how resources will be allocated and organized) rather than on the essential service that is provided through special education—i.e., problem solving. This author's contention is that special education serves its clients by functioning as the problem-solving component of our general education system. The various administrative arrangements and procedural mechanisms that seem to define special education—resource programs, special classes, individualized education programs, due process procedures, etc.— tend to obscure the fact that special education is funded to provide solutions to a specific set of school-based social problems that are associated with the intellectual and personal development of children.

Whereas general education programs are designed to foster the development of all children, special education programs are designed to foster the development of students for whom general education programs are unsuccessful. Special education exists, then, because all general education programs fail to educate effectively some portion of the students assigned to those classroom programs. Special education seeks to solve the problem of how to provide more effective programs for individual students who are not served adequately in their education by the core, or mainstream, educational program.

THE NATURE OF MILD HANDICAPS

Historically, special education resources have been provided on the assumption that there is a subset of the population called "handicapped" who have a right to specialized treatment beyond that provided through the general education program. The values underlying that position are that providing these special additional educational services is (1) necessary in a humane and caring society and (2) economically beneficial to society in the long run. Since precious public resources are allocated on the basis of the concept "handicapped," we must first define who are the handicapped persons eligible for specialized educational services.

To draw a conclusion regarding who is eligible for the additional resources provided through special education, it is useful to consider the distinctions among the terms "impairment," "disability," and "handicap." Since the CBM procedures used in special education problem solving have been applied primarily to describe the behavior of mildly handicapped students, the discussion here is limited to the nature and definition of "mildly handicapped."

In the problem-solving approach presented here, the term "handicap" is defined broadly as a problem that exists when the environmental demands placed on an individual exceed that individual's current capabilities for meeting those demands. In this view, students who are required to answer questions about a story that they have been assigned to read are handicapped if they cannot read that story. Similarly, the student required to write a brief story who does not have the necessary writing skills is handicapped; the child who must complete mathematical story problems but cannot do simple computation is handicapped; the teacher who is required to provide an education for a diverse group of 25 students who does not have the required organizational and management skills to effect the achievement of all students is handicapped; and the person who wishes to sing in a choir and cannot carry a tune is handicapped. Thus, when successful adaptation to the environment requires abilities that the individual does not possess, the individual is handicapped.

The term "disability" is often used in connection with the definition of the term handicap. Although differences exist regarding what is meant by the term, general agreement exists that "disability" refers to a condition of the individual that limits, or interferes with, that person's efforts to meet current and future environmental demands. In the field of special education, the term "disability" historically has been reserved for those performance limitations that had a clearly identifiable organic basis. The organic basis was called an "impairment." In school settings, for example, students whose disabilities in reading, writing, and arithmetic were attributable to impaired vision or hearing were those whose handicaps (i.e., their failure to be able to answer teacher questions because of their skill deficiencies) were thought to justify the expenditure of additional money for special education programs. As the field of special education developed, additional disability conditions were identified, each with a strong advocate group arguing for the special and organic nature of the disability condition, and as the economic costs of increased numbers of students identified as "handicapped" have escalated, competition for limited special education resources has become fierce.

One result of the increased competition has been an effort on the part of some policy advocates to require that the organic basis, or impairment, causing any disability clearly be established prior to allocation of services to the individual possessing those disabilities. Inherent in this "impairment" approach are the assumptions that (1) the same disability may have different causes, (2) some students' disabilities are organically based, (3) other students' disabilities are not organically based, and (4) the distinction can clearly be made between the organic and nonorganic basis of the disability. A related assumption in the impairment approach to determining disabilities is that the nonorganically based disabilities are the result of environmental factors such as an impoverished home, inadequate parenting, or poor quality of instruction. The advantages of the impairment position appear to be primarily practical and economic. On the surface, to make such a distinction should enable us to delimit special education allocations to a smaller subset of those disabled students who are handicapped in their efforts to meet the demands placed on them by the schools.

The problem with taking the position that some students' disabilities are organically based and others are environmentally based is that it is inconsistent with the interactionist view regarding human development that prevails in contemporary psychology. The interactionist view holds that the development of all human abilities is a product of the interplay between biological characteristics and environmental experiences rather than the simple outcome of one or the other. Further, although separate estimates of the respective contributions of the environment and biology to development are sometimes made (Plomin & Daniels, 1987), such estimates are very gross and preliminary and refer only to the determinants of general traits such as intelligence and temperament rather than to the development of specific skills. Finally, very little is known regarding the degree to which environmental experiences cumulatively affect the relative contributions of biology and environment in the acquisition of ability. Early learning success may be more a function of inherited characteristics, but the cumulative effects of learning specific skills may diminish the importance of any initial advantage.

When the prevailing interactionist view is applied to the problem of identifying those students whose handicaps are the result of organically based disabilities, it becomes clear that such a problem is not now, nor may ever be, solvable. Such a position may be factually incorrect. At present, it is certainly technically impossible to measure the degree to which human abilities and disabilities are the result of organic impairment.

In the case of certain specific organic conditions (e.g., sensory impairments), the causal connection between the disability and the organic condition is clear. In such cases, the apparent connection is sufficient justification for providing services. Sensory impairments, orthopedic impairments, and brain injuries, for example, would provide the necessary and sufficient basis for establishing the right to special education. Since this issue extends beyond that group of students typically referred to as "mildly handicapped," not much is discussed here in regard to these connections. However, it would be well to remember that individuals with similar degrees of such impairments often differ markedly with respect to scope of their disabilities and the magnitude of their handicaps. Thus, two people who are legally blind but with different environmental histories may differ markedly with respect to the abilities they possess for meeting the demands placed on them by their environments, both inside and outside of school.

PERSON-CENTERED VERSUS SITUATION-CENTERED PROBLEMS

If special education is to function as a problem-solving mechanism in the general education system, the nature of the problem to be solved by special education must be clear. The foregoing discussion regarding disabilities and handicaps provides a useful framework within which to consider the problems to be solved by special education. As is clear from that discussion, disabilities are centered within the individual; that is, they can be defined in terms of the individual's skill deficiencies or lack of competence. Since the term "disability" literally means "that which disables," it is clear that just as an illness disables a person with respect to carrying out ordinary living activities, a deficiency in reading disables a person from carrying out ordinary intellectual activities required both inside and outside of school. Since this disability resides within the individual, we can say that it is person-centered.

In contrast to person-centered disabilities, handicaps are situation-centered. Handicaps can only be defined in terms of the relationship between what a person *can* do and what a person *must* do to succeed in a given environment. Therefore, whether or not a handicap exists depends not only on what a person can do but also on the performance that is required of the individual for successful adaptation to the environment. A lack of reading skill becomes a handicap only when success in the environment requires a level of reading skill not possessed by the individual. A reading disability becomes a handicap when the teacher requires the student to answer questions based on text material or when a person is required to read directions in order to assemble a bicycle. Since handicaps exist in the relationship between the individual and the environment, they are situation-centered rather than person-centered. Handicaps, then, are ecologically defined since they can be described only in terms of the network of social and physical environmental relationships of which the individual is a part.

Handicaps as Performance Discrepancies

A useful approach to describing mild handicaps is to specify the difference between the performance required of an individual in a given situation and the performance actually achieved by the individual in that situation. In school settings, this difference is identified by examining the requirements set by the teacher in making assignments and giving grades and comparing those requirements with measures of the student's level of accomplishment when he/she attempts to meet those requirements. Mager and Pipe (1970) used the term "performance discrepancy" to refer to this difference between the level of performance one expects and the level of performance one observes when analyzing performance problems. In the problem-solving approach presented here, performance discrepancies, regardless of their etiology, are the handicaps that must be overcome if the individual is to be perceived as successful by both school and society.

Defining Mildly Handicapped

The position taken in this book is that the problems special education should be required to solve are the significant performance discrepancies faced by a relatively small proportion of students who do not meet the reasonable performance expectations set in the general educational program of their schools. The assumption is made that by provision of additional support services to modify their programs, this subset of students will eventually be able to meet the same minimum academic requirements set for all students to attain a high school diploma. It is not necessary to modify the educational goals for these "mildly handicapped" students. Instead, what is required is an intensification of efforts to reduce the handicaps to a point at which they do not prevent successful completion of schooling. By definition, then, mild handicaps are distinguishable from moderate handicaps in that it is unreasonable to expect students with moderate handicaps to achieve the ordinary requirements for high school graduation.

Defining Special Education Problems

Handicaps have been defined here as situation-centered performance discrepancies. Although such a definition is useful, two problems must be addressed: (1) the situation-specific nature of problems and (2) the myriad of expectations that define performance as discrepant.

Since performance discrepancies can only be defined with reference to specific situations, it is common to find that someone can be handicapped in one situation (e.g., the school) but not handicapped in another (e.g., the job). Students who do not compute well enough to complete word problems successfully in their math class may experience no difficulty in accomplishing the computation required for working in a fast-food restaurant. Indeed, most of us who might have been poor math students in school are not mathematically handicapped in our daily lives. It is also common to find that a student whose academic performance is acceptable in one school or classroom may be discrepant from the expectations of another teacher in a different school or classroom although he/she is performing at the same level. For example, a student whose performance in reading might have led to eligibility for special education services in a high-achieving suburban school district might be placed in a top reading group and not be referred to special education in a low-achieving urban school. Even within the same school, a student's behavior is likely to be judged differently by different teachers from one grade to the next. Indeed, Balow and Rubin (1978) found that being identified as possessing a significant behavior problem by at least one teacher is quite normal during a student's elementary school years. The situational nature of handicaps makes it difficult to determine whether or not a particular handicap represents a problem sufficiently important to solve through allocation of precious special education resources.

A second difficulty one encounters when using the performance discrepancy approach to defining special education problems is the myriad of academic and social behavioral expectations placed on students in school. In general, teachers expect (1) compliance to reasonable requests, (2) attention and participation in class, (3) completion of independent classwork and homework, (4) self-direction on projects, and (5) development of accuracy and fluency on a variety of curriculum skills. When the specific expectations within this general set of expectations are identified, however, some seem clearly less important than others. In the area of curriculum expectations in reading, for example, no empirical justification can be provided for requiring the established levels of performance on curriculum-embedded basal mastery tests before allowing a student to move ahead to new levels in the curriculum. In fact, evidence exists that the tests accompanying many reading series are not sufficiently reliable and valid to make such decisions (Tindal et al., 1985). In contrast, there is evidence that requiring students to spend more time reading will yield higher achievement (Leinhardt, Zigmond, & Cooley, 1981). Given both the myriad of expectations and the situational nature of many handicaps, it becomes clear that some set of criteria, or system, must be used to establish whether a handicap is important enough to resolve through special education.

The Role of Cultural Imperatives

A useful framework for considering the distinction between important and unimportant handicaps is provided by the concept of the "cultural imperative" (Reynolds & Birch, 1977). Cultural imperatives are the implicit or explicit standards of conduct or performance imposed on all who would be members of a culture. An example of a cultural imperative in American society that occasionally produces conflict is the requirement that all citizens speak English. Some imperatives are codified in law, such as the paying of taxes; others such as the expectation that adults should be independent are sanctioned socially but are not legally required. One significant role played by the public schools in America is the inculcation of many socially sanctioned but not legally required cultural imperatives. Although controversy exists over what constitutes the cultural imperatives to be transmitted by our schools (cf., Hirsch, 1987), the most commonly identified set of imperatives fall into the category designated as "basic skills." Although differing viewpoints exist regarding what is encompassed by the term "basic skills," functional literacy in reading, written expression, and arithmetic are commonly identified as basic and required of all children.

Cultural imperatives may be contrasted with cultural electives— those activities, proficiencies, and standards of conduct that are valued within a society but are not required of all members. Playing a musical instrument, for example, is widely valued, but it is not required for acceptance into our society. Therefore, although music is offered and encouraged in the schools, instrumental skill in music typically is not required for promotion through the grades. The distinction between reading as a cultural imperative and the playing of a musical instrument as a cultural elective readily translates into the distinction between a handicap important enough to be considered a problem requiring special education and a handicap insufficiently important to allocate the resources used in special education problem solving.

The Centrality of "Difference" in All Problem Identification

The distinction between cultural imperatives and cultural electives only provides a partial basis for identifying those problems important enough for special education services. A second criterion that must be added is the size of the difference between what a culture requires in its imperatives and what a member must do to be considered "at risk" for violating cultural expectations. More directly, by how much must an individual's performance differ from the performance standards set by the culture for him or her to be considered mildly handicapped? From an empirical, psychological point of view, the answer is to be found in the normative behavior of the members of that culture. In this view, establishing important differences requires development of empirical norms that largely, but not exclusively, determine the performance standards imposed by the culture. Rightly or wrongly, the cultural press is for performance standards derived from the performance of same-aged peers.

Commercially developed norm-referenced tests rest on the assumption that the standards for performance in reading, written expression, and arithmetic that are established for students at any time during the school year are best derived from the typical performance of same-aged cohorts at that time during the school year. Arguments might be made that this is inappropriate. The perspective taken here, however, is that, at the present time, the difference that defines a student as mildly handicapped is a measured *normative* difference in learning from cultural imperatives. The failure to perform those imperatives as required is observed and responded to by the significant others in a student's environment—particularly teachers and parents. Teachers and parents typically become concerned when they perceive that a student's performance is widely different from peer performance, and as a result, they may initiate action toward resolving this difference.*

Since handicaps are situational, judgments of "sufficient difference" reside in, and are conditioned by, the local social contexts within which a student's behavior occurs. This perspective means that teachers do not make judgments of sufficient difference based only on the universal norms of the culture; instead, their judgments are also based on the behavior of the students in classrooms and schools within which they are working. This point is important to remember when policies are developed regarding who should receive special education service, and it is a point that is reintroduced in later chapters when the use of CBM procedures to identify and place students in special education programs is described.

Whereas it is true that the standards for acceptable performance in a society derive, largely, from the normative behavior of its members, it would be incorrect to assume that the performance standards for cultural imperatives derive solely from normative behavior. The periodic calls for reform in our schools clearly illustrate the use of standards other than those derived from prevailing norms. These calls for reform typically occur when performance norms are viewed by the society as markedly decreasing or inferior to the norms in other cultures. In the early 1980s, for example, the schools were sharply criticized for apparent decreases in the national averages on the Scholastic Aptitude Test (SAT). Further, considerable alarm was created by evidence that students from Japan were superior in their mathematical performance to students in the United States. The result was a call for the raising of performance standards on cultural imperatives above those that had been derived from the normative performance of students graduating from high school. As previously noted, teacher standards also vary from cultural norms because these judgments are influenced by the performance of students in specific classrooms. Thus, teachers in schools with large pro-

---

*It is worth noting here that both parent's and teacher's causal attributions regarding the basis for differences in performance relate to whether or not they will initiate action to solve a significant performance discrepancy. As a result of a cross-cultural study, Gordon (1987) concludes that American teachers and parents attribute differences to inherent ability rather than to efforts to learn made by the student. Asian teachers and parents hold the opposite view and, instead of accepting these differences as Americans do, act to produce greater efforts to learn on the part of low-achieving students.

portions of low-achieving children are likely to establish implicit and explicit performance standards that are much lower than those derived from the general population of students in the United States. The effects on academic achievement of low performance standards have been sufficiently clarified through research so that the expectation of higher levels of performance is viewed as a primary characteristic of effective schools (Minnesota Educational Effectiveness Project, 1987).

In sum, special education has been described here as that component of the schools that should solve the individual educational problems that inevitably occur in the context of programs provided through general education. These problems, called performance discrepancies, become important when significant differences in performance exist on cultural imperatives, and these significant performance discrepancies define mild handicaps. A final point to be made about special education relates to the nature of the problem-solving efforts organized and managed by special education.

Special Education as Hypothesis Testing

The literature on problem solving in human affairs is convincing in its demonstration that effective problem solving requires that the problem solvers generate many possible plans of action prior to attempting problem solution (Johnson & Johnson, 1982). Alternative plans of action are important for two reasons: first, selection of a "best solution" requires consideration of alternatives; second, problems frequently are not solved successfully through application of the first attempt at problem solution. The successful problem solver is one who can devise many strategies to solve the same problem. Solving special education problems requires the same consideration and application of alternatives. Indeed, in the ideal case, the development of a student's individual education plan (IEP) is an illustration of group problem solving in which alternative possible programs are considered. From this perspective, the IEP represents a particular plan of action or reform in a student's program that will reduce the magnitude of important performance discrepancies that have been identified. The process of special education problem solving, then, becomes the consideration, selection, and application of these various solution hypotheses intended to eliminate students' handicaps.

The problem-solving procedures described throughout this

volume are derived from single-case, time-series research designs (Glass, Willson, & Gottman, 1975). The use of research procedures in special education problem solving adds systematic empirical testing of alternative hypotheses or reforms in students' programs. The predicted gain from applying scientific procedures to solving special education problems is that the continuous and systematic application of these procedures will produce cumulative improvements in the educational programs of individual mildly handicapped students. If such improvements occur, they should increase the likelihood that student handicaps will be reduced sufficiently to enable full and unsupported participation in the mainstream society.

The empirical problem-solving approach presented here is derived from the proposition advanced almost 20 years ago by Donald Campbell in his presidential address to the American Psychological Association. In that address, he proposed that reforms in human affairs be treated as experiments whose effects need to be tested rather than assumed (Campbell, 1969). When that proposition is applied to special education, it becomes clear that the reforms in students' programs brought about through special education require careful empirical testing. Empirically testing reforms helps to ensure that the precious resources allocated through special education do indeed lead to the reduction of those problems for which these resources are allocated.

A SPECIAL EDUCATION PROBLEM-SOLVING MODEL

Systematic efforts in problem solving require the organization and sequencing of activities—the use of a problem-solving model. The problem-solving model used with curriculum-based measurement involves five steps: (1) identifying the problem to be solved, (2) defining the problem, (3) considering alternative solutions, (4) implementing alternative solutions, and (5) determining when the problem has been solved. The problem-solving steps correspond to the IDEAL problem-solving model described by Bransford and Stein (1984) and correspond quite closely to the administrative steps that occur in providing special education services. Although the basic steps are common to most problem-solving models, what makes the approach presented here different from the others is the reliance on a data base created through use of a specific set of measurement procedures to collect time series data as an aid to evaluating problem-solving efforts. Table 1.1 illustrates the relationships among each problem-solving step, the curriculum-based measurement data, and the evaluation activities that correspond to each problem-solving step. In the model, measurement is distinguished from evaluation to clarify that the purpose of measurement is numerical description, whereas the purpose of evaluation is decision. In measuring performance discrepancies, we seek to provide an objective, reliable, and precise data base that can contribute to decision making. Our evaluations of those discrepancies involve consideration of data, but they also require a weighing of values, laws, regulations, resources, and the probable personal and social consequences of selecting different courses of action. The data from measurement can inform and direct decisions, but they neither dictate nor determine those decisions.

TABLE 1.1 A Data-Based Problem-Solving Model

Problem-solving steps (administrative steps)	Measurement activities	Evaluation activities
1. Problem identification (screening/ referral)	Observing and recording student performance on cultural imperatives	Deciding that a performance problem exists
2. Problem definition (assessment and eligibility determination)	Describing the differences between actual and expected performance	Deciding what discrepancies, if any, are important enough to be solved
3. Considering exploring alternative solutions (IEP[a] goal setting intervention planning)	Estimating probable performance improvements and costs associated with different solutions	Selecting the program reform (i.e., solution hypothesis) to be tested
4. Implementing solutions, monitoring of IEP progress towards IEP objectives, (periodic/annual reviews)	Monitoring implementation of IEP and student performance changes	Determining whether the solution attempt should be continued or revised
5. Problem solution (program termination)	Describing the difference between actual and expected performance	Deciding that existing discrepancies, if any, are not important, and program (IEP) may be terminated

[a]Individual Education Program

As can be seen by inspecting Table 1.1, the problem-solving steps, measurement activities, and evaluation activities correspond to the steps usually identified as requirements in providing special education service to students through PL 94–142. Typically, students are referred to special education; the referral is screened to determine the need for further assessment; if appropriate, assessment for determining eligibility follows; if the subject is eligible for service as handicapped, an IEP is developed including annual goals, short-term objectives, evaluation procedures, and the service to be provided; the IEP is then implemented, and student progress toward IEP goals monitored; finally, the success of an IEP is reviewed periodically and annually to determine program success.

Although the problem-solving model presented in Table 1.1 corresponds quite closely to the procedures used by school districts to comply with law and regulation, it should be pointed out that the term "eligibility" associated with step 2 of the problem-solving model can be misleading. In traditional special education programming, determination of "eligibility" means that a decision must be made to justify the expenditure of special education monies to solve the problem that has been defined.

Current rules and regulations are not always precise and tend to be controversial regarding how "eligibility" determinations are to be made in special education (cf. Galagan, 1985). In many instances, the rules that allow eligibility determination may have very little to do with the plans of action, or "treatments," that might be generated to address the basis for the initial referral (Heller, Holtzman, & Messick, 1982). In fact, it may be clearer to view the current rules and regulations as procedures for establishing the right to use special education monies in the same way that rules are traditionally used in "third-party" payment systems (e.g., insurance carriers and welfare systems) to establish whether or not third-party payments can be made. In the case of Medicare and Medicaid, for example, the rules regarding eligibility are independent of the medical problem to be solved. Rather, the rules require that eligibility be based on the person's age and other personal circumstances. The medical problems, themselves, exist irrespective of whether eligibility for insurance payments is established. Similarly, in education, if current federal and state rules are applied, important performance discrepancies can be identified and defined that cannot be solved using special education money.

The operation of special education as a third-party payer and the problem it creates is illustrated in the following example. Suppose a beginning third-grade student who cannot even read stories from the preprimer is referred to special education. In many states the child will not be eligible for special education unless an IQ test score is obtained that is either above the 16th percentile or below the 3rd percentile. In those states that require a comparison of IQ and achievement test scores, the child will be eligible as learning disabled if the obtained IQ is normal, whereas if the IQ were sufficiently lower than normal, the child would be eligible as mentally handicapped. If this child's IQ score were to fall between "normal" and "retarded," the classification might only be that of a "slow learner" who is ineligible for special education. It should be emphasized that the magnitude of this student's reading disability is the same regardless of the obtained IQ score. Further, the personal, social, and economic consequences of continued failure to learn to read will be the same whether the student is labeled learning disabled, mentally handicapped, or slow learner. From this example, it should be apparent that present regulations are directed toward resolving when payment should be provided and not toward determining the existence of important problems.

A more practical approach than the one dictated by current law and regulation would be an approach that would permit expenditure of additional monies to solve any important performance discrepancy without regard for the presumed cause of that discrepancy. Such an approach would significantly reduce costs associated with determining eligibility as now required by law and regulation. Although this is an issue well worth debate, its resolution is unnecessary for successful use of CBM and should not distract us from the application of the problem-solving model presented here.

Standardized Curriculum-Based Measurement Procedures

As will become evident throughout the remainder of this volume, the curriculum-based measurement procedures advocated for use in resolving the performance problems of mildly handicapped students comprise a set of specific measurement procedures that can be applied to quantify student performance in reading, written expression, spelling, and arithmetic. These procedures are the product of a systematic research and development program that established the technical adequacy of the data collected through applying these measurement procedures to student performance (cf. Deno, 1985, 1986). The fact that these procedures are standardized rather than *ad hoc* assures a data base for individual problem solving that is sufficiently reliable and valid. The issue of technical adequacy is especially important when comparisons are made between an individual student and the performance of that student's peers. The reliability and validity of data are also important when comparisons are made of the same student's performance at different times such as before, during, and after various attempts to solve a problem. In general, any time the data obtained from two or more measurements are compared, the reliability of those measurements is an important issue. Further, any time a question arises as to whether or not a performance discrepancy is important, the validity of a particular measurement or set of measurements must be established. It is not possible to be confident that any of the myriad performance discrepancies that could be identified through measuring a student's performance on somewhat arbitrarily selected curriculum tasks would be sufficiently important to attempt problem solution. The following chapters will clearly reveal that the scope and rigor of data collection efforts by those people using curriculum-based measurement in special education problem solving provide them with a reliable and valid data base for decision making.

REFERENCES

Balow, B., & Rubin, R. (1978). Prevalence of teacher identified behavior problems: A longitudinal study. *Exceptional Children, 45,* 102–111.

Bransford, J. D., & Stein, B. S. (1984). *The IDEAL problem solver.* New York: W. H. Freeman.

Campbell, D. T. (1969). Reforms as experiments. *American Psychologist, 24,* 409–429.

Deno, E. (1970). Special education as developmental capital. *Exceptional Children, 37*(3), 229–237.

Deno, S. L. (1985). Curriculum-based measurement: The emerging alternative. *Exceptional Children, 52*(3), 219–232.

Deno, S. L. (1986). Formative evaluation of individual student programs: A new role for school psychologists. *School Psychology Review, 15*(3), 348–374.

Galagan, J. E. (1985). Psychoeducational testing: Turn out the light, the party's over. *Exceptional Children, 52*(3), 288–299.

Glass, G. V., Willson, L. L., & Gottman, J. M. (1975). *Design and analysis of time series experiments.* Boulder, CO: Laboratory of Educational Research, University of Colorado.

Gordon, B. (1987). Cultural comparisons of schooling. *Educational Researcher, 16*(6), 4–7.

Heller, K. A., Holtzman, W., & Messick, S. (1982). *Placing children in special education: A strategy for equity.* Washington: National Academy Press.

Hirsch, E. D. (1987). *Cultural literacy.* Boston: Houghton Mifflin.

Johnson, D. W., & Johnson, F. P. (1982). *Joining together* (2nd ed.). Englewood Cliffs, NJ: Prentice-Hall.

Leinhardt, G., Zigmond, N., & Cooley, W. (1981). Reading instruction and its effects. *American Educational Research Journal, 18*(3), 343–361.

Mager, R. F., & Pipe, P. (1970). *Analyzing performance problems.* Belmont, CA: Frason Publishers.

Minnesota Educational Effectiveness Project. (1987). *Program components.* St Paul: Minnesota State Department of Education, Technical Report.

Plomin, R., & Daniels, D. (1987). Why are children in the same family so different from one another? *Behavioral and Brain Sciences, 10,* 1–60.

Reynolds, M. C., & Birch, J. W. (1977). *Teaching exceptional children in all America's schools.* Reston, VA: Council for Exceptional Children.

Tindal, G., Fuchs, L., Fuchs, D., Shinn, M., Deno, S. L., & Germann, G. (1985). Empirical validation of criterion referenced tests. *Journal of Educational Research, 78,* 203–209.

2

A Curriculum-Based Measurement Approach to Assessing Academic Performance: What It Is and Why Do It

Douglas B. Marston

As discussed in Chapter 1, there exists a serious need to examine alternative testing models for making educational decisions. In this chapter, this need is documented from the perspective that the traditional model has failed education in two major ways, from the technical level and from a social policy level. Curriculum-based measurement procedures are proposed to redress some of the issues in these domains.

PROBLEMS WITH TRADITIONAL ASSESSMENT AND THE FAILURE OF THE PSYCHOMETRIC MODEL

Why is there a need for an alternative set of assessment procedures/devices? A look at the *Ninth Mental Measurements Yearbook* (Mitchell, 1985) shows literally thousands of published psychological and educational tests that can be used by educators. Given the plethora of assessment devices, it could be asked fairly why some of these assessment devices are not suitable for making the kinds of decisions school psychologists are asked to make and why a new set of procedures is required.

Although individual published tests can be useful for specific, albeit limited, and important purposes (e.g., screening, program evaluations), traditional published tests are problematic for special education decision making for two general reasons. First, at the measurement and psychometric level, there is great concern about the technical adequacy (i.e., reliability, validity, norms) of these measures. Second, at the social policy level, many of these tests have not been proven to be useful in decision making because of legal and practical issues.

At the Measurement–Psychometric Level

For any set of assessment procedures, a primary concern is the quality of their technical adequacy. The guidelines established by the American Psychological Association, the American Educational Research Association, and the National Council on Measurement in Education (1985) state that all tests used in education and psychology must be valid, reliable, and, if they are to be used in a norm-referenced manner, have adequate normative data. In their review of assessment procedures used in special education, Salvia and Ysseldyke (1982) listed a number of frequently used tests that were not technically adequate with respect to validity, reliability, and quality of the normative sample. Similar tables have been developed by Berk (1984). Salvia and Ysseldyke (1982) cautioned educators about the use of technically inadequate tests and warned that they would adversely impact the psychoeducational decision-making process in special education.

These issues are compounded when the use of these devices with handicapped children is considered. Fuchs, Fuchs, Benowitz, and Berringer (1987) surveyed 27 frequently used published intelligence and achievement tests and examined how often handicapped students were included in (1) the standardization sample, (2) the development of test items, and (3) the establishment of indices of reliability and validity. Only five of the 27 tests "provided specific percentages to indicate handicapped children's participation in some aspect of test development" (Fuchs et al., 1987).

Many educators might argue that although technically problematic tests in the area of education exist, well-trained school psychologists, specialists, and teachers would not use such tests. Unfortunately, research data indicate otherwise. A group of 159 educators, psychologists, and specialists were asked to review the case histories of children referred to special education and then select assessment procedures necessary for identification and program planning (Ysseldyke, Algozzine, Regan, & Potter, 1980). Analysis of those instruments chosen for assessment indicated that 67% of the selected tests lacked sufficient evidence for validity, 59% lacked acceptable standards for reliability, and 66% did not have adequately described norms. Assuming the results generalize to practice, Ysseldyke et al. (1980) concluded that there is a significant degree of uncertainty introduced into the special education decision-making system. As a result, the overall impact on the delivery of services to handicapped children may be problematic.

Content Validity

A second problem associated with traditional tests is the content validity of these measures. Unfortunately, many school psychologists and special education teachers too often fail to differentiate their use of published achievement tests in practice. Erroneously, achievement tests are treated equally and are used interchangeably. Unfortunately, the decisions "based upon these instruments are subject to the biases of the test administered as well as the curriculum employed" (Shapiro, 1987).

Prevailing professional opinions recognize that published achievement tests frequently fail to sample adequately the curriculum taught the student. The various achievement tests available to educators differentially sample the many curricula used in our schools. Without careful attention to the potential testing–teaching overlap (or lack thereof), test scores do not truly index pupil skill level, since they may not measure what the child has learned. A number of published studies have documented this concern. In an analysis of teaching content between five standardized tests of reading achievement and five reading curricula, Jenkins and Pany (1978) found that expected grade scores for a given test varied widely as a function of the reading curriculum the child would be taught. They estimated that second-grade pupils taught in Houghton-Mifflin would score at the 3.2 grade level on the Peabody Individual Achievement Test (Dunn & Markwardt, 1970), but only 2.2 when instructed in Ginn 360.

More recently, the Jenkins and Pany (1978) study was replicated by Shapiro and Derr (1987). Based on five basal reading series and four individually administered achievement tests, they found that the overlap between the curriculum and test word lists differed markedly. Their findings support Jenkins and Pany's results that the scores obtained on the tests could vary according to the specific test administered and the particular reading curriculum in which the student was receiving instruction. For example, the standard scores (mean of 100, standard deviation of 15) on the achievement tests across curricula that would be attained hypothetically for first-grade students ranged from 6 on the Woodcock Reading Mastery (Woodcock, 1973) to 16 for the PIAT; first graders instructed in *Keys to Reading* (Houghton-Mifflin) would be expected to score at the 68th percentile on the PIAT compared to the 27th percentile if they were receiving reading instruction in Ginn 720. Shapiro and Derr (1987) also found that the overlap between the curricula and the basal reading series decreased with successive grade levels: fewer word matches between the curricula and test word lists existed after the third grade.

Concern about testing–teaching overlap is not confined to reading, however. Freeman et al. (1983) obtained similar results in math. Their study showed that the proportion of topics covered in math achievement tests given more than cursory treatment in specific math curricula never exceeded 50% and could be as low as 20%. Nor is the problem constrained to the initial testing of students. Critically, the problem of testing–teaching overlap is confounded when students' progress is assessed. Eaton and Lovitt (1972) examined the progress of learning-disabled students over a 9-month period using two different reading tests. These authors found several pupils in a class made significant gains on the Wide Range Achievement Test (WRAT) (Jastak & Jastak, 1978) but not on the Metropolitan Achievement Test (MAT) (Durost, Bixler, Wrightstone, Prescott, & Balow, 1971). Conversely, several pupils in the same class made significant progress on the MAT, whereas testing with the WRAT demonstrated little evidence of improvement. One of the conclusions that was offered is that because standardized achievement tests fail to sample adequately the content of what the teacher is teaching, measuring change on the tests may be invalid, and the conclusions drawn about progress may be erroneous.

Irrelevance for Instructional Planning

Special education teachers also question the usefulness of traditional published tests in planning and improving students' instructional programs. Thurlow and Ysseldyke (1982) examined this point by asking 200 school psychologists and special education teachers how instructionally useful published norm-referenced tests were. Given a list of commonly administered tests, including the Wechsler Intelligence Scale for Children–Revised (WISC-R) (Wechsler, 1974), Bender Visual Motor Gestalt (Koppitz, 1963), and the WRAT, 100 school psychologists rated the measures with respect to their utility for instructional planning. Seventy-two percent of the school psychologists reported that the WISC-R was helpful, 64% endorsed the Bender, and 80% rated the WRAT as aiding program planning. When 100 special education resource teachers were asked to evaluate the same list of tests, a different perspective emerged: only 10% considered the Bender as instructionally relevant, 30% rated the WISC-R as useful during the IEP planning process, and 10% said the WRAT contributed to developing effective instructional plans. Two related conclusions can be drawn from this study. First, school psychologists and special education teachers should communicate with each other about the relevance of test information and instructional planning. Second, teachers of the handicapped may need alternative assessment procedures from those traditionally provided to help plan instruction.

Indirect Assessment: Selection-Type Responses

Another problem with traditional assessment devices is their reliance on test items that measure skills indirectly. Although this problem is most apparent when intelligence tests are used to plan academic programs, this same problem is often true with achievement tests. The primary obstacle is the response format(s) of the test. Few achievement tests actually require the student to perform the behavior of concern. Instead of reading or writing, they may require selection-type items (Popham & Baker, 1970) such as matching (e.g., PIAT Spelling), pointing to (e.g., Woodcock-Johnson reading comprehension), or crossing out correct or incorrect items. Multiple-choice items on reading comprehension tests are a good example. After a child reads a passage on a standardized test, he/she is often confronted with a question followed by several possible answers or solutions.

The advantages of these types of items are (1) their ease of scoring, (2) their conservation of time, (3) good interscorer reliability, and (4) promotion of a generally representative test because of the increased possibility of large numbers of items

(Popham & Baker, 1970). Disadvantages of selected-response items are that they take an extensive period of time to prepare if the test has not been constructed by others and that guessing may confound a student's score. Additionally, selection-type responses are related to how well a child "takes tests" and even to "fine-motor coordination." Since all of these variables may factor into the student's reading score, for example, and impact the final score, school psychologists need to ask if this is the most direct measure of reading. Further, the most extreme limitation of these types of responses is that they provide little or no information on why a student earns a particular score. This point is exemplified by Howell and Kaplan (1980), who maintain that "it is not readily obvious why a student made a mistake . . . because she is not required to produce anything except a pencil mark on the answer sheet" (p. 21). Thus, all that is learned is that the student did or did not answer the item correctly, no reason can be seen why the problem was answered as it was. It is the task analysis of errors that contributes invaluable information for instructional planning and placement.

Fluency Not Considered

Contributing to the limitations of selection type responses is the consequent ignoring of the importance of fluency of responding. For example, most published tests of reading achievement fail to consider fluency during assessment (Ysseldyke & Marston, 1982). Yet fluency is one of the principal building blocks on which reading skills are built. Samuels (1979) notes that reading fluency is intertwined with comprehension and recommends the use of repeated readings to build fluency. As he states, "teachers may wonder what role reading comprehension plays in the rereading method. Repeated reading is a meaningful task in that the students are reading interesting material in context. Comprehension may be poor with the first reading of the text, but with each additional rereading, the student is better able to comprehend because the decoding barrier to comprehension is overcome gradually. As less attention is required for decoding, more attention becomes available for comprehension. Thus, rereading both builds fluency and enhances comprehension" (Samuels, 1979).

The importance of fluency of responding is described further by White and Haring (1980), who point out that children who work slowly, despite being accurate, have not actually mastered a skill. However, students who may be less accurate in their work but can finish it more quickly may have attained mastery.

The significance of fluency in reading has led the Commission on Reading (1985) to remark in their report, *A Nation of Readers,* that "readers must be able to decode words quickly and accurately so that this process can coordinate fluidly with the process of constructing the meaning of the text" and that "more comprehensive assessments of reading are needed. Standardized tests do not provide a deep assessment of reading comprehension and should be supplemented with observations of reading fluency. . . ."

The Inadequacy of the Pre–Post Test Design to Evaluate Change

Traditionally, school psychologists and special educators have relied on the pre–post test design for the purpose of measuring change in student learning. This type of analysis is inappropriate for four reasons. First, measurement experts have challenged the notion that published norm-referenced tests are adequately designed to measure learner outcome. Hively and Reynolds (1975) pointed out that most standardized, norm-referenced tests have been developed with the explicit purpose of *measuring individual differences,* a perspective that does not easily lend itself to the evaluation of pupil growth. Carver (1974) refers to this emphasis on measuring pupil differences and abilities as the *psychometric* dimension of testing. In his review, he cites the necessity for designing *edumetric* tests, procedures that measure student learning: "Because the psychometric dimension has been focused on traditionally, many standardized tests are used to measure gain or growth without being developed or evaluated from an edumetric standpoint. The danger of this approach is that the psychometrically developed tests may not be sensitive to gain when in fact there is gain" (p. 518). As a result of their designed purpose of measuring individual differences, published norm-referenced tests are often insensitive to pupil growth. Although students actually may be improving, the design of the test precludes the demonstration of learning.

Marston, Fuchs, and Deno (1986) demonstrated this point in a comparison of CBM procedures and published norm-referenced achievement tests. Over a 16-week period, students grew significantly on CBM reading measures; growth was far less evident on the published measures of reading comprehension and vocabulary. Importantly, teacher judgment of pupil growth was in much greater agreement with CBM than with the published tests. Similar results were reported by Marston and Magnusson (1985) over a 10-week period.

Second, as reported earlier, pre–post gains are confounded when the testing–teaching overlap is uncertain. In a classic study by Eaton and Lovitt (1972), the progress of learning-disabled (LD) children from fall to spring was inconsistent across two achievement tests. Such fluctuations are probably best attributed to the poor match between test content and actual instruction (Jenkins & Pany, 1978).

A third reason that published achievement tests fail to capture student progress accurately is the type of scores used most frequently, grade and age equivalents. Though used frequently, they have been an anathema in all major assessment texts because of their poor statistical properties and misrepresentation of level of student performance. In actuality, they are a form of percentile rank that communicates very poorly. Like percentile ranks themselves, they provide indices of relative standing that provide little or no information about what a child can or cannot do. They can only be interpreted in the context of how the normative group is performing.

A fourth problem is the unreliability of measuring pre–post gain for individual students. Cronbach and Furby (1970) note that individual difference scores over time tend to be very unstable, making it difficult to assess student improvement.

Finally, the very nature of the *frequency* of the pre–post evaluation is problematic. The types of approaches are summative in nature; they can be used only to say what has or has not occurred. The data are too late to be used formatively (i.e., to make substantive revisions in ineffective instructional programs).

At the Implementation/Social Policy Level

Cost of Current Assessment

Among the primary criticisms, educators have concluded that the assessment process is expensive and time-consuming (Mirkin, 1980; Ysseldyke, Thurlow, et al., 1983). The expense of eligibility determination often is estimated to exceed the costs of educating the child (Ysseldyke, Thurlow, et al., 1983). For example, in a national survey of directors of special education, Poland, Thurlow,

Ysseldyke, and Mirkin (1982) reported the average reimbursement for educating a mildly handicapped student to be $2300 per
year. In contrast, they also found that the time spent in assessment
for determining eligibility was substantial, ranging from 4.5 to 156
hours. At the high end, the cost of assessment was estimated to be
over $3000 per child, a figure clearly in excess of available
reimbursement rates. The extensive time expenditure is evident
particularly in the case of school psychologists who, depending on
the survey cited, spend 50%–75% of their time in the mildly
handicapped eligibility determination process (Goldwasser, Meyers, Christenson, & Graden, 1984; Hughes, 1979). According to
Goldwasser et al. (1984), school psychologists devote approximately 70% of their day to testing students for eligibility decisions. At
28 hours per 40-hour work week, this is quite an expensive en-
deavor. In a survey of school psychologists conducted by Smith
(1984), psychologists indicated that they desired a significant
reduction of their assessment responsibilities with a corresponding
increase in intervention and consultation endeavors.

If time and expense were the only issue, it seems as if traditional
eligibility assessment practices would be defensible. In fact, it
could be argued that the decision to label a student should be
made on extensive data that do not come cheaply. Other important criticisms of current procedures, however, have been levied.
In many cases, the specific procedures used to certify students as
handicapped have undergone criticism as being discriminatory
(Boyan, 1985; Sewell, 1981), and as a result, they have ended up
being the subject of court rulings (Sandoval, 1987).

Limited Use of the Data in Team Decision Making

Perhaps no criticism of traditional assessment and decision making
has been greater than that of its inconsistency with respect to
individual student's special education eligibility. This inconsistency
generally takes two forms: (1) the lack of consistent decision-
making criteria on a state-to-state, district-to-district, and often
school-to-school basis and (2) the failure of multidisciplinary teams
to adhere to the decision indicated by the specific eligibility
criteria. In point of fact, in many cases, schools often disregard the
assessment data and place students in special education who do
not meet the eligibility criteria (Ysseldyke, Algozzine, Richey, &
Graden, 1982). That is, as evidenced by Ysseldyke, Algozinne,

Richey, et al. (1982), when investigators examine the degree to which the actual eligibility decision made by the multidisciplinary team matches the expected decision according to the Federal definition of learning disabilities, the decision can be characterized as having "very little to do with the data collected on the students" (p. 78). In several of the observational studies conducted by this research team it was apparent that team decisions frequently did not conform to the test results presented at the team meeting. In other words, teams were ignoring published test data in favor of other information deemed more important. Why do teams not utilize the data for decision purposes? The most probable explanation is that they judge such data as limited in usefulness. Even where stringent eligibility criteria are in place, a significant number of students are placed who may not meet the standards or vice versa. This finding was exemplified in a study reported by Wilson (1985). When a discrepancy of 1.5 standard errors of measurement between IQ and achievement scores was used, 26% of the students placed into special education programs did not meet this criterion.

Definitional Ambiguities Regarding Handicaps and Lack of Differential Diagnosis

Standardized test data have been shown to be not terribly useful in making clear decisions about pupil placement in special education, often referred to as differential diagnosis. Ysseldyke, Algozzine, Shinn, and McGue (1982) studied the use of the WISC-R, the Woodcock–Johnson Psychoeducational Battery, the PIAT, the WRAT, and the Developmental Test of Visual-Motor Integration (Beery & Buktenica, 1967) in differentiating LD pupils from non-LD students. Their data show that on standardized tests of achievement and ability there is over 90% overlap between these two groups. Similar findings have been demonstrated at secondary school levels (Warner, Schumaker, Alley, & Deshler, 1980). These results suggest that, on an individual basis, it would be practically impossible to make a differential diagnosis with any confidence. Such outcomes have been demonstrated by Epps, Ysseldyke, and McGue (1984). They presented extensive case study data to teachers, school psychologists, and engineering students naive to special education practices. The groups were no different in their accuracies (or inaccuracies) in matching test data to students' labels. The use of published tests for identifying learning-disabled students is confounded in studies of normal students (i.e., students not considered as having learning problems at various grades). Many normal students could be identified as learning disabled (Ysseldyke, Algozzine, & Epps, 1983). For example, when a significant discrepancy between ability and achievement was defined as a 10-point difference between the WISC-R full-scale IQ and standard scores from subtests of the Woodcock–Johnson Achievement test and the PIAT, 65% of normal students met the criterion. When learning disability was defined as a 1-standard-deviation discrepancy between these same measures, 25% of normal students met the criterion. Using 17 different definitions of learning disabilities found in the literature, Ysseldyke, Algozzine, et al. (1983) found that 88% of normal students were identified by at least one of the definitions, and 4% of school-identified learning-disabled students were not identified by any of the definitions.

Legal Trends and the Need for an Alternative Assessment Model

If there is a common theme to be found in education-related litigation in this nation's courts, that theme would revolve around the appropriate use of tests. *Larry P. v. Riles* (1979), *Diana v. State Board of Education* (1970), and *Hobson v. Hansen* (1967) all point to problems inherent in the standardized testing process and verify the need for examining alternatives.

As a result of these cases and others, statutory laws have been targeted directly or indirectly at the assessment process (Forness & Kavale, 1987). For example, the Protection in Evaluation Procedures (PEP) guidelines in Public Law (PL) 94-142 (Section 615-5C) pronounce that "Procedures to assure that testing and evaluation materials and procedures utilized for the purposes of evaluation and placement of handicapped children will be selected and administered so as not to be racially or culturally discriminatory." Further, as specified in the *Federal Register,* August 23, 1977 (p. 42474), "Tests that are used must have been validated for the specific purpose for which they are used."

Despite these legislative assurances, Galagan (1985) argued that many current assessment procedures do follow the requirements of PL 94-142. He wrote, "the pervasive employment of these legally deficient instruments loses all rationale in the face of emerging CBA measures. These measures are child- and curriculum-directed, entailing a genuine individual focus, and thus are more capable of identifying and addressing the specific educational needs of children and therefore the legal requirements of the Education for all Handicapped Children Act."

Continuity across Special Education Decisions

Salvia and Ysseldyke (1985) maintain that good assessment practice extends beyond identification decisions. Educators, they state, must concern themselves with a continuum of psychoeducational decisions, including (1) screening, (2) eligibility/identification, (3) program planning, (4) pupil progress monitoring, and (5) program evaluation. In the traditional special education decision-making approach, a "mixing apples and oranges" format is employed. That is, different assessment devices collected by different persons are used for making each of the different educational decisions (Ysseldyke & Thurlow, 1984). For example, when making screening decisions, the regular classroom teacher or principal often relies on group-administered tests such as the Stanford Achievement Test or the Metropolitan Achievement Test. In the eligibility determination process, testing responsibility typically shifts to the school psychologist who places a heavy reliance on individually administered, norm-referenced tests as required by PL 94-142. When instructional programs are planned, special education teachers become more involved. They base their plans on a variety of assessment procedures including norm-referenced achievement tests, "diagnostic tests," the placement tests that accompany curricula, and informal testing. Traditional assessment practices for monitoring progress are documented less well. Fuchs, Fuchs, and Warren (1982) found that most monitoring of progress is made with teachers' subjective opinions, accompanied by pre–post, individually administered, published achievement tests. Finally, the area of program evaluation is usually saturated with all types of tests found in the above categories. In addition to this wide assortment of tests used across decision areas, the educator is confronted with a diverse set of test scores, including (1) raw scores, (2) percentile ranks, (3) deciles, (4) stanines, (5) standard scores, (6) age and grade equivalents, (7) mastery scores, and (8) developmental quotients.

Given this state of affairs, it is obvious a common metric or decision-making standard does not exist across all of these significant decision areas. The basis of decision making, therefore, changes as a function of the interaction of the data collected and the decision to be made. It is argued that such unevenness and diversity in tests and test scores across decision areas is detrimental to the decision making that occurs.

ESSENTIAL FEATURES AND ADVANTAGES OF THE CBM MODEL

Curriculum-based measures are premised on a number of salient characteristics that were considered desirable for monitoring student progress (Jenkins, Deno, & Mirkin, 1979). Among the criteria were that the measure(s) had to be (1) tied to a students' curricula, (2) of short duration to facilitate frequent administration by teachers/educators, (3) capable of having many multiple forms, (4) inexpensive to produce in terms of time in production and in expense, and (5) sensitive to the improvement of students' achievement over time. Another necessary characteristic was the identification of academic behaviors in the basic skill content areas that educators could measure reliably and validly. During the late 1970s and early 1980s, the research of Stanley Deno and Phyllis Mirkin at the University of Minnesota's Institute for research on Learning Disabilities (IRLD) focused on the field testing of the technical adequacy of a number of potential measures of curricular performance that had been published in the professional literature in an attempt to validate their use in decision making. The following measures were identified as curriculum-based measures of student achievement:

1. In the area of reading, counting the number of words a student reads correctly from either a basal reader or word list in a 1-minute interval.
2. In the area of written expression, counting the number of words or letters written during a 3-minute interval, given either a story starter or topic sentence.
3. In spelling, counting the number of correct letter sequences (White & Haring, 1980) or words spelled correctly during a 2-minute interval, given words dictated every 7 seconds.
4. In the area of math, counting the number of correctly written digits during a 2-minute interval from grade-level computational problems.

Other salient characteristics of CBM include its focus on direct, repeated measurement of student performance in the curriculum using production-type responses. Importantly, CBM provides data that are useful across the range of special education decisions including screening and eligibility determination.

Direct Measurement of Performance in the Curriculum

A significant characteristic of CBM is the emphasis on direct measurement. Shapiro (1987) defines direct measurement as representing "the behavior of interest to be assessed by noting its occurrence. As such, the data are empirically verifiable and do not require any inferences from observations to other behaviors" (p. 31). As pointed out earlier, most published achievement tests typically rely on indirect measurement of pupil skills with respect to the source of test items and the student response formats. As detailed by Deno (1985, 1986), CBM is based on a major premise that assessment and decision making are curriculum referenced. That is, a student's performance on a test should indicate the student's level of competence in the local school curriculum. The content validity of the measure is critical. For example, in CBM, reading measures are developed using passages drawn from the pupil's basal reading series. Similarly, spelling words are drawn from the instructional domain that the student is to learn.

Production-Type Responses

In CBM, assessment focuses on measurement of *observable* pupil skills to increase the utility of the assessment process. Students must actually perform the behavior of concern, by writing or by saying. For example, in reading, rather than ask students to read passages silently and then to write answers on pencil–paper tasks, the examiner listens to the child read aloud and conducts the assessment on this sample of behavior. As described by Popham and Baker (1970), production-type responses have a number of advantages over selection-type responses. First, they often allow the assessor to observe the process the student used to derive the answer correctly or incorrectly. This latter piece of information is critical to error analysis and instructional planning. Second, they allow students to "display creative or novel solutions to problems" (Popham & Baker, 1970). Third, the stimulus materials are produced in less time than other teacher-constructed tests. Production-type responses do have one major liability; they may be more time-consuming and less reliable to score than tests with selection-type responses. This potential disadvantage, however, is not always inherent in specific measures.

CBM Technical Adequacy

Research on the development of reliable and valid measures of student performance in the basic skill curricula proceeded in five steps. First, an extensive analysis of the literature was conducted to identify potential measures. Second, the research team convened in multiple sessions to review the potential measures with respect to the established criteria. Third, those measures that appeared to meet many of the criteria were field tested for their criterion-related validity. Fourth, reliability studies were conducted. Fifth, studies of logistics of measurement (e.g., length of testing interval, size of the measurement domain) were implemented.

Reading Validity

The initial CBM validity study in reading was conducted by Deno, Mirkin, and Chiang (1982). Deno, Mirkin, et al. (1982) identified five measures of reading that potentially could be employed to monitor students' progress on a frequent basis. These measures required students to:

1. Read aloud stories from their basal reader (passage reading).
2. Read aloud lists of words randomly selected from the pupil's basal reader (isolated word lists).
3. Read aloud words underlined in a story from his/her basal reader (reading in context).
4. Supply words that had been deleted from stories from their basal reader (Cloze comprehension procedure).
5. Give the meaning of words selected from the basal reader story (word meaning).

These measures then were correlated with criterion tests of reading—generally accepted, published norm-referenced tests. The criterion measures selected for the first validity study were the Stanford Diagnostic Reading Test (Karlsen, Madden, & Gardner, 1975), the Woodcock Reading Mastery Test (Woodcock, 1973), and the Reading Comprehension subtest from the Peabody Individual Achievement Test (Dunn & Markwardt, 1970). Deno, Mirkin, et al. (1982) found that listening to students read aloud from their basal reader for 1 minute was a valid measure of reading skill. Correlation coefficients ranged from .73 to .91, with most coefficients above .80. Since that initial study, a number of other criterion-related validity studies have been conducted. The authors, dates, subjects, criterion measures, and results of these studies are presented in Table 2.1.

In these latter studies, correlation coefficients between a student's oral reading from the basal reader and different published measures of global reading skills ranged from .63 to .90, again with most coefficients being above .80. Correlation coefficients between oral reading fluency and the subtests on these global measures were somewhat lower although still adequate, ranging from .53 to .91. Ten of the 20 coefficients exceeded .80. Lower correlation values for some of these subtests would be expected because of their lower reliabilities.

Further criterion-related validity was demonstrated between reading fluency measures and four different basal reading series' criterion-referenced mastery tests. Correlations between the total test scores and reading fluency measures (both passages and word lists) ranged from .57 to .86 with four of eight coefficients being above .80. In this comparison, the degree to which the curriculum-based measures were correlated with the basal mastery tests was directly proportional to those measures' correlation with more global measures of reading proficiency. In other words, the curriculum-based reading measures shared more variance with those basal mastery tests that were correlated highly with general measures of reading skills than with those that were less related to other measures of reading ability. This finding provides additional support for the criterion-related validity of curriculum-based reading measures as a predictor of global reading proficiency.

With the basal mastery tests used as a criterion, reading from passages was found to be more highly related to test performance than was reading from word lists. The median correlation between reading orally from passages and the mastery tests was .84, whereas the median correlation between reading words from a list and the mastery tests was .76 (only one of four coefficients reached .80). Thus, in addition to being an excellent predictor of generalized reading ability, 1-minute measures of students' reading of passages from their reading books appears to be a better predictor of their success in the curriculum than their performance on reading a word list.

In addition to standardized tests of reading competency and

TABLE 2.1 Summary of Validity Studies for Curriculum-Based Measures of Reading

Study	Subjects	Criterion measure	Results
Deno, Mirkin, et al., 1982 (word lists)	18 regular education/15 special education, grades 1 to 5	Stanford Diagnostic Reading Test (SDRT)	.76
		WRMT Word Identification subtest	.91
		WRMT Word Comprehension subtest	.83
		Cloze	.87
		Word meaning	.90
(passages)		Stanford Diagnostic Reading Test (SDRT)	.73
		WRMT Word Identification subtest	.87
		WRMT Word Comprehension subtest	.82
		Cloze	.89
		Word meaning	.81
Deno, Mirkin, et al., 1982 (word lists)	43 regular education/23 special education, grades 1 to 6	SAT Phonetic Analysis subtest	.68–.71 (range)
		SAT Reading Comprehension subtest	
		Inferential Comprehension	.74–.75 (range)
		Literal Comprehension	.68–.71 (range)
		PIAT Reading Comprehension subtest	.76–.78 (range)
		Cloze	.84–.86 (range)
		Word meaning	.60–.63 (range)
(passages)		SAT Phonetic Analysis subtest	.71
		SAT Reading Comprehension subtest	
		Inferential Comprehension	.80
		Literal Comprehension	.78
		PIAT Reading Comprehension subtest	.76
		Cloze	.86–.87 (range)
		Word meaning	.56–.57 (range)

Study	Sample	Measure	
Fuchs, Tindal, & Deno, 1984 (third-grade word lists)	45 students, grades 3 to 6: 27 regular education, 18 mildly handicapped	Cloze Comprehension task	.84
		Word meaning task	.60
(sixth-grade word lists)	45 students, grades 3 to 6: 27 regular education, 18 mildly handicapped	Cloze Comprehension task	.86
		Word meaning task	.63
(third-grade passages)	45 students, grades 3 to 6: 27 regular education, 18 mildly handicapped	Cloze Comprehension task	.86
		Word meaning task	.57
sixth-grade passages)	45 students, grades 3 to 6: 27 regular education, 18 mildly handicapped	Cloze Comprehension task	.87
		Word meaning task	.56
Marston, 1982 (third-grade word list)	83 low-achieving students, grades 3 to 6, who earned low scores (below 15th percentile) on a written expression task	SAT Vocabulary subtest	.85
		SAT Comprehension subtest	.72
		SAT Word Study	.74
		SAT total test score	.84
Marston, 1982 (grade-level word list)	57 low-achieving students, grades 4 to 6, who earned low scores (below 15th percentile) on a written expression task	SAT Vocabulary subtest	.53
		SAT Comprehension subtest	.54
		SAT Word Study	.65
		SAT total test score	.63
Marston & Deno, 1982 (grade-level basal reader)	26 regular education students in grade 3	Science Research Associates Vocabulary	.80
		Science Research Associates Comprehension	.80
		SAT Vocabulary subtest	.59
		SAT Reading Words subtest	.84
		SAT Comprehension subtest	.88
		SAT Word Study subtest	.84
		SAT total reading test	.90
		Classroom teacher's holistic rating	.77

(continued)

TABLE 2.1 (continued)

Study	Subjects	Criterion measure	Results
Fuchs, Fuchs, & Maxwell, 1982	35 mildly handicapped students: 27 LD, 7 SED, 1 EMR; grades 4 to 8	SAT Reading Comprehension subtest SAT Word Study subtest Written and oral recall measures Cloze comprehension measure	.91 .80 .75 (mean) .63–.86 (range) .75 (mean) .62–.85 (range)
G. Tindal, M. R. Shinn & L. S. Fuchs, (unpublished data) (grade-level basal reader)	90 regular education students, grades 4–6; within grades converted to z-scores	Question-answering measure Science Research Associates Vocabulary Science Research Associates Comprehension	.84 .67 .59
M. R. Shinn, M. Upson, & S. Stein (unpublished raw data) (grade-level basal reader)	61 regular education students, grade 2	CAT Vocabulary (fall) CAT Comp (fall) Harcourt, Brace, Jovanovich Basal Mastery Comprehension (spring)	.69 (spring CBM) .75 (spring CBM) .59 (spring CBM)
Fuchs & Deno 1981 (grade-level basal reader)	15 special education/23 Chapter 1, and 53 regular education, grades 1 to 6	Woodcock Reading Mastery (WRM) WRM Word Identification (raw score) WRM Passage Comprehension (raw score) Teacher judgment (placement)	.82 (mean) .85 (mean) .86 (median)

Study	Test	Correlation
Tindal, Shinn, Fuchs, Fuchs, Deno, & German 1983 47 regular education students, grade 6 (passages) (word list)	Houghton Mifflin Mastery total test	.65
	Decoding composite	.47
	Comprehension composite	.66
	Reference/study skills composite	.68
	Houghton Mifflin Mastery total test	.57
	Decoding composite	.36
	Comprehension composite	.55
	Reference/study skills composite	.57
Fuchs, Tindal, Shinn, et al., 1983 47 regular education students, grade 5 (passages) (word list)	Ginn 720 Mastery total test	.83
	Comprehension subtests	.72
	Vocabulary subtests	.85
	Decoding subtests	.65
	Study Skills subtests	.58
	Ginn 720 Mastery total test	.80
	Comprehension subtests	.69
	Vocabulary subtests	.81
	Decoding subtests	.65
	Study Skills subtests	.52
Tindal, Fuchs, Fuchs, Shinn, Deno, Germann 1983 25 regular education students, grade 4 (passages)	Scott Foresman total test	.84
	Word Identification Scale	.70
	Comprehension Scale	.70
	Study and Research Scale	.76
	Literary Understanding/Appreciation	.55

(continued)

TABLE 2.1 (*continued*)

Study	Subjects	Criterion measure	Results
(word list)		Scott Foresman total test	.77
		Word Identification Scale	.42
		Comprehension Scale	.52
		Study and Research Scale	.73
		Literary Understanding/Appreciation	.58
Fuchs, Tindal, Fuchs, et al., 1983 (passages)	21 regular education students, grade 4	Holt Basic Reading Series Management	
		Program Level 13 total test	.86
		Comprehension/Literary Skills	.79
		Decoding/Encoding Skills	.75
		Language Skills	.46
		Study Skills	.58
(word list)		Holt Basic Reading Series Management	
		Program Level 13 total test	.75
		Comprehension/Literary Skills	.75
		Decoding/Encoding Skills	.64
		Language Skills	.55
		Study Skills	.57

basal mastery tests of student achievement, teacher judgment was used to demonstrate further oral reading fluency's utility as a measure of generalized reading skill. Two studies examined the relationship between CBM reading measures and teachers' holistic rating of the students' reading ability. In the first study, Fuchs and Deno (1981) found that for a group of 91 first through sixth graders sampled from both regular and special education settings, reading fluency measures were highly related to teachers' judgment of student reading proficiency (median $r = .86$). In a study by Marston and Deno (1982), the relationship between oral reading fluency and teacher holistic ratings of reading skills was significantly greater than teacher ratings with published achievement tests and their actual reading placement in the curriculum. These findings provide further evidence of reading fluency's criterion-related validity. In addition, they allude to curriculum-based measurement's great utility for helping to make pupil placement, program-planning, and program evaluation decisions.

An important reading validity study was completed recently. Fuchs, Fuchs, and Maxwell (1988), provided further data with respect to oral reading fluency as a valid measure of reading comprehension. Using 70 mildly handicapped middle school students as subjects, they examined the relations between more traditional measures of comprehension, question answering, recall (written and oral), and Cloze with oral reading fluency and two reading subtests (Reading Comprehension and Word Study Skills) of the Stanford Achievement Test. Their results indicated that oral reading fluency correlated most highly with the criterion measures (.89). In fact, the correlations were significantly greater than that of the second higher measure, written recall (range from .66 to .82).

Currently, G. Tindal, M. R. Shinn, and V. Collins (unpublished data) are attempting to examine the relationship of reading fluency, decoding, and comprehension using covariance structure analysis and causal modeling. Their preliminary results suggest that, as expected given the extensive concurrent validity studies, oral reading fluency contributes significantly to a model of reading and may be as valid a measure of comprehension as decoding. This latter finding would be in direct contradiction to how educators have viewed oral reading fluency, that is, as synonymous with rapid decoding.

In addition to investigating criterion-related validity, Deno and his colleagues studied the construct validity of the measures using three major strategies: discriminant validity, longitudinal studies of reading growth, and treatment validity. To investigate the discriminant validity of the reading measure, the degree to which the reading measure distinguished intact groups that differed in their reading skills theoretically was studied. Deno, Marston, Shinn, and Tindal (1983) established the discriminant validity of 1-minute oral reading samples when they reliably differentiated learning disabled from Chapter I and regular education first-, second-, and third-grade students. This finding was replicated by Shinn and Marston (1985), who found that words read aloud differentiated regular education students, pupils served in Chapter I, and mildly handicapped students with learning difficulties. Marston, Tindal, and Deno (1983) demonstrated that CBM procedures predicted LD classification as well as traditional measures of aptitude–achievement discrepancy.

The validation of the reading measure was also demonstrated in the study of sensitivity to growth. Because a valid measure of reading would be expected to show growth as student skills improve, a series of studies were initiated. A cross-sectional study of oral reading fluency across grades 1 through 6 in a sample of 550 elementary students showed reliable gains (Deno, Marston, Mirkin, et al., 1982). Marston, Fuchs, and Deno (1986) examined the short-term reading progress of students across 10-week and 16-week intervals with both standardized reading tests and CBM procedures. Although both approaches identified student improvement, the CBM procedures (1) delineated greater growth in the reading performance of students and (2) correlated much more closely with teacher perceptions of individual student improvement.

Reading Reliability

The IRLD investigators also examined the reliability of CBM procedures. These studies, by author, subject, type of reliability, and results, are summarized in Table 2.2.

Reliability estimates for CBM reading measures were determined using three methods, all of which yielded impressive findings. First, test–retest reliability estimates were examined using test–retest intervals of 1 to 10 weeks. Reliability coefficients ranged from .82 to .97 with most estimates being above .90. Second, parallel form estimates were also excellent, ranging from .84 to .96, again with most correlations above .90. Finally, interrat-

TABLE 2.2. Summary of Reliability Studies for Curriculum-Based Measures of Reading

Study	Subjects	Type of reliability	Results
Marston, 1982 (Grade 3 word list)	83 students who scored below 15th percentile in written expression, grades 3 to 6	Test–retest (10 weeks) 10 parallel forms, 1 week apart	.90 .90 (mean) .85–.96 (range)
(Grade-level list)		Test–retest (10 weeks) 10 parallel forms, 1 week apart	.82 .91 (mean) .84–.94 (range)
Shinn, 1981 (Grade-level list)	71 LD and low-achieving students, grade 5	Test–retest (5 weeks) 4 parallel forms, 1 week apart	.90 .91 (median) .89–.94 (range)
Tindal, Germann, et al., 1983 (passages)	30 regular education students, grade 5	Test–retest (2 weeks)	.97
Tindal, Germann, et al., 1983 (passages)	110 regular education students, grade 4	2 parallel forms at same time	.94
Tindal, Marston, et al., 1983 (passages)	566 randomly selected students, grades 1 to 6	Test–retest (10 weeks) Alternate form (1 week) Interjudge agreement	.92 .89 .99

er agreement coefficients were examined and found to be outstanding at .99. Taken together these findings provide compelling evidence of the reading measures reliability of CBM.

Spelling Validity

In three initial spelling validation studies, Deno, Mirkin, Lowry, and Kuehnle (1980) examined the extent to which (1) words spelled correctly (2) words spelled incorrectly, (3) correct letter sequences written, and (4) incorrect letter sequences written correlated with other spelling criterion measures such as the Spelling subtest of the Stanford Achievement Test (Madden, Gardner, Rudman, Karlsen, & Merwin, 1973), the Test of Written Spelling (Larsen & Hammill, 1976), and the Spelling subtest from the Peabody Individual Achievement Test (Dunn & Markwardt, 1970). The number of correct and incorrect letter sequences is a scoring procedure, devised by White and Haring (1980), that was designed to be more sensitive to changes in spelling skills. In the first study, subjects were administered three word lists of varying difficulty and the Test of Written Spelling. In the second study, four varying word lists were used, and the Spelling Subtests of the Peabody Individual Achievement Test (Dunn & Markwardt, 1970) served as the criterion measure. In the third study, again four word lists were used, and the criterion measure was the Spelling subtest of the Stanford Achievement Test. Words were dictated to students at set intervals of time (every 10 seconds) for 3 minutes. The results of the Deno, Mirkin, Lowry, et al. study (1980) are presented in Table 2.3. They found that both the number of words spelled correctly and correct letter sequences were valid measures of spelling skills. Correlations with the criterion measures in this study ranged from .80 to .96. In addition, it was determined that 1-, 2-, and 3-minute-long samples provided equivalent results in terms of the validity coefficients. Additional follow-up validity studies are presented in Table 2.3.

Across studies, correlations with the criterion spelling measures were all above .80, regardless of whether the spelling sample was scored for the number of words or correct letter sequences written. The validity coefficients ranged from .81 to .95.

Various forms of construct validity for the CBM spelling measures have also been demonstrated. The discriminant validity of the spelling measures was established in two studies by Shinn and Marston (1985) and Shinn, Ysseldyke, Deno, and Tindal (1986).

TABLE 2.3. Summary of Validity Studies for Curricular-Based Measures of Spelling by Scoring Metric

Study	Subjects	Criterion measure	Words correct	Correct letter sequences
Deno, Mirkin, Lowry, et al., 1980 (3 word lists of varying difficulty)	15 LD and 27 regular education students, grades 2 to 6	Test of Written Spelling	.95 (median) .87–.96 (range)	.93 (median) .86–.99 (range)
Deno, Mirkin, Lowry, et al., 1980 (4 word lists of varying difficulty)	10 LD and 35 regular education students, grades 2 to 6	Peabody Individual Achievement Test	.88 (median) .83–.94 (range)	.84 (median) .80–.90 (range)
Deno, Mirkin, Lowry, et al., 1980 (4 word lists of varying difficulty)	29 LD and 32 regular education students, grades 2 to 5	Stanford Achievement Spelling subtest	.88 (median) .83–.89 (range)	.86 (median) .80–.86 (range)
Marston, 1982	57 low-achieving students, grades 4 to 6, who earned low scores (below 15th percentile) on a written expression task	Stanford Achievement Spelling subtest	.87	.81

Shinn and Marston (1985) evaluated the degree that CBM spelling measures differentiated 209 fourth-, fifth-, and sixth-grade students placed in mildly handicapped, Chapter I, and regular-education-only programs. Results of the study indicated that CBM spelling measures reliably distinguished the three groups regardless of whether the metric of analysis was the number of correct words or correct letter sequences spelled. Mildly handicapped students scored significantly lower than Chapter I students, who scored significantly lower than students who received only regular education instruction. These results were replicated by Shinn et al. (1986) in their contrast of 34 learning-disabled and 37 low-achieving students over a 5-week time period in spelling.

Further evidence of construct validity was shown by two studies (Deno, Marston, Mirkin, et al., 1982; Marston, Lowry, Deno, & Mirkin, 1981) that demonstrated that the performance on CBM spelling measures improves as students progress through the school year and receive more spelling instruction. In both studies, student CBM spelling performance showed significant growth across the school year for regular education elementary-aged students.

Spelling Reliability

The results of a series of reliability studies in spelling using the number of words spelled correctly and correct letter sequences are presented in Table 2.4.

When we compare reliability data across these studies, we find the test–retest coefficients for words spelled correctly to be high (.85–.94). Similar results are obtained when the metric is the number of correct letter sequences (.83–.93). The magnitudes of these coefficients are much the same when reliability is examined using a parallel form paradigm. Reliability estimates range from .72 to .96 for words spelled correctly and from .80 to .97 for correct letter sequences. The average interscorer reliability coefficients were .99 and .91 for words and correct letter sequences, respectively.

Written Expression Validity

The initial investigation of CBM written expression measures consisted of a series of three concurrent validity studies (Deno, Mirkin, & Marston, 1980). These studies explored the validity of

TABLE 2.4. Summary of Reliability Studies of Curriculum-Based Spelling Measures by Type of Scoring System

Study	Subjects	Type of reliability	Words correct	Correct letter sequences
Marston, 1982	83 3rd–6th graders, who scored below 15th percentile in written expression	Test–retest (10 weeks) 10 parallel forms, 1 week apart	.87 .80 (mean) .72–.88 (range)	.92 .87 (mean) .73–.92 (range)
Shinn, 1981	71 LD and low-achieving 5th graders	Test–retest (5 weeks) 4 parallel forms, 1 week apart	.85 .85 (median) .82–.92 (range)	.83 .84 (median) .80–.92 (range)
Tindal, Germann, et al., 1983	30 regular education 5th graders	Test–retest (2 weeks)	.94	.93
Tindal, Germann, et al., 1983	30 regular education 4th graders	2 parallel forms at same time	.82	.82
Tindal, Marston, et al., 1983	566 regular education students, grades 1–6	Test–retest (20 weeks) 2 parallel forms at same time	.91 .96	.86 .97
		Interjudge scoring	.99	.91

(1) number of words written, (2) number of words spelled correctly, (3) number of correct letter sequences, (4) number of mature word choices, (5) number of large words written, and (5) Hunt's (1966) average *t*-unit length as potential measures. All six measures were correlated with the following criterion measures: the Test of Written Language (Hammill & Larsen, 1978), the Developmental Sentence Scoring System (Lee & Canter, 1971), and the Language subtest of the Stanford Achievement Test (Madden et al., 1978). A subsequent study (Deno, Marston, & Mirkin, 1982) replicated these procedures by researching the correlations between the same six production and the criterion measures listed above.

The results of these two studies indicated that total words written, words spelled correctly, correct letter sequences, and mature words were highly related to the criterion measures. In addition, the study by Deno, Mirkin, and Marston (1980) demonstrated that compositions could be written using story starters, picture stimuli, or topic sentence and that the length of the written samples could range from 2 to 5 minutes with equivalent results. A review of these and other concurrent validity studies is presented in Table 2.5.

Correlations between total words written and the criteria measures ranged from .41 to .84. In addition to published achievement measures, Videen, Deno, and Marston (1982) also used teacher holistic ratings of writing skill as a criterion measure. Their study indicated that total words written was a valid measure of written expression (correlation of .85) when compared to this standard. Of the two studies that reported lower validity coefficients (i.e., below .50), the subjects in one study (Marston, 1982) were comprised of low-achieving students who performed below the 15th percentile on written expression. With this restricted range of scores, a lower correlation coefficient is not unexpected.

As presented in Table 2.5, the correlations between words spelled correctly and the criterion measures ranged from .45 to .92. Most coefficients were above .70. The range of correlations for correct letter sequences was narrower, .57–.86, although fewer studies have been conducted using this measure.

Other studies have investigated the use of CBM written expression measures to differentiate the academic performance of intact groups of students. Marston, Mirkin, and Deno (1984) compared a screening and referral procedure that used weekly measurement in written expression (writing samples scored according to number of words written) to a traditional teacher procedure. This study

TABLE 2.5. Summary of Validity Studies for Curriculum-Based Measures of Written Expression by Scoring Metric

Study	Subjects	Criterion measure	Total words	Words correct	Correct letter sequence
Deno, Mirkin, & Marston, 1980	16 LD students, 16 regular education students, grades 3 to 6	Test of Written Language total test	.63	.67	—
Deno, Mirkin, & Marston, 1980	4 LD students, 24 regular education students, grades 3 to 6	Test of Written Language subtests	.41–.70 (range)	.45–.67 (range)	—
		Test of Written Language total test	.81	.79	—
		Stanford Achievement Test	.65	.69	—
Deno, Mirkin, & Marston, 1980	31 LD students, 51 regular education students, grade 3 to 6	Developmental Sentence Scoring	.84	.84	.78
Deno, Marston, & Mirkin, 1982	44 LD students, 86 regular education students, grades 3 to 6	Test of Written Language total test	.75	.80	.85
		Test of Written Language subtests	.58–.69 (range)	.60–.71 (range)	.57–.74 (range)
		Developmental Scoring Sentence	.84	.76	.86
		Stanford Achievement Test	.62		
Marston, 1982	57 low-achieving students, grades 4 to 6, who earned low scores (below 15th percentile) on a written expression task	SAT Language subtest	.47	.64	.61
Videen et al., 1982	50 regular education students, grades 3 to 6	Test of Written Language	.66	.92	—
		Developmental Sentence Scoring	.51	.52	—
		Teacher holistic rating	.85	.84	—

demonstrated that the use of repeated curriculum-based measures resulted in referral rates that approximated the same number of students for special education. The CBM referrals also appear to negate the influence of biasing factors such as gender and social behavior.

Shinn and Marston (1985) further established that consistent differences between the academic performance of mildly handicapped students and those students in regular education or receiving Chapter I services could be determined using CBM procedures. A comparison of these three groups of students showed that there were significant performance discrepancies in written expression between the mildly handicapped students and those students in regular education or receiving Chapter I services in grades 4 to 6. No significant differences were found between regular education students and students receiving Chapter I services in grades 5 and 6.

Student growth in written expression on a longitudinal basis was studied by Marston et al. (1981) and Deno, Marston, Mirkin, et al. (1982). In both studies, elementary students in grades 1 to 6 significantly increased in total words written, total words written correctly, and number of correct letter sequences during the course of the academic school year. Examination of shorter-term progress over 10- and 16-week periods showed significant gains for total words written (Marston et al., 1986).

Written Expression Reliability

The results of a number of reliability studies in the written expression measure for total words written, words spelled correctly, and correct letter sequences are summarized in Table 2.6.

The reliability estimates for CBM procedures in written expression were determined using test–retest, parallel forms, and interrater agreement. Test–retest reliability estimates were as follows: .42 to .69 for total words written; .62 to .81 for words spelled correctly; and .51 to .86 for correct letter sequences. Parallel form estimates ranged from .51 to .84, with most coefficients above .70, for total words written. Reliability correlation coefficients were reported at .41 to .85 and from .64 to .96 for words spelled correctly and for correct letter sequences, respectively. The interrater scoring agreement for the three measures was high with a mean of .98.

In general, the reliability estimates of single administrations of

TABLE 2.6. Summary of Reliability Studies of Curriculum-Based Written Expression Measures by Type of Scoring System

Study	Subjects	Type of reliability	Total words	Words correct	Correct letter sequence
Marston, 1982	83 3rd–6th graders who scored below 15th percentile in written expression	Test–retest (10 weeks) 10 parallel forms, 1 week apart	.42 .58 (mean) .42–.71 (range)	.46 .59 (mean) .41–.73 (range)	.51 .64 (mean) .49–.73 (range)
		Parallel forms determined by averaging 3 weekly measures	.70–.84 (range)	—	—
Marston & Deno, 1981	28 LD students, grades 1 to 6	Test–retest (1 day)	.91	.81	.92
Marston & Deno, 1981	161 students, grades 1 to 6	Test–retest (3 weeks) 2 parallel forms, same day	.64 .95	.62 .95	.70 .96
Marston & Deno, 1981	105 students, grades 1 to 6	Split-half, minutes (2+5) with (3+4) Split-half, minutes (2+4) with (3+5)	.99 .99	.96 .97	.98 .99
Marston & Deno, 1981	4 trained graduate students with samples from 20 pupils, grades 1 to 6	Cronbach's *alpha* Interrater scoring	.87 .98 (mean)	.70 .98 (mean)	.87 .99 (mean)
Shinn, 1981	71 LD and low-achieving 5th graders	Test–retest (5 weeks)	.69	.73	.71
		4 parallel forms, 1 week apart	.59 (median) .51–.71 (range)	.59 (median) .52–.74 (range)	.64 (median) .55–.73 (range)

(continued)

TABLE 2.6 *(continued)*

Study	Subjects	Type of reliability	Total words	Words correct	Correct letter sequence
Tindal, Germann, et al., 1983	60 regular education 5th graders	Test–retest (2 weeks)	.56	—	—
Tindal, Germann, et al., 1983	60 regular education 4th graders	2 parallel forms at same time	.70	—	—
Tindal, Marston, et al., 1983	566 regular education students, grades 1 to 6	Test–retest (6 months)	.70	—	.86
		2 sets of 2 parallel forms, same time	.73 (mean)	—	.93 (mean)
Tindal, Marston, et al., 1983	4 trained graduate students, 566 regular education pupils, grades 1 to 6	Interrater scoring	.98 (mean)	—	.98 (mean)
Fuchs, Deno, et al., 1983	78 3rd to 6th graders who scored below 15th percentile in written expression	10 parallel forms, 1 week apart			
		2 samples		.55	—
		4 samples	—	.72	—
		6 samples	—	.85	—
		8 samples	—	.88	—
		10 samples	—	.89	—

CBM written expression measures are lower than the other academic areas. To improve the reliability of the measures, Fuchs, Deno, and Marston (1983) investigated the effects of aggregation on the reliability of curriculum-based measures using the number of words spelled correctly. Based on the administration of 10 parallel forms 1 week apart, their results indicated that stability coefficients increased from .55 for two samples to .89 for 10 samples. This study provides evidence that aggregating over samples and forms greatly improves the test reliability.

Math Validity

Investigators in the Pine County Special Education Cooperative (Tindal, Germann, & Deno, 1983) and the Minneapolis Public Schools (Skiba, Magnusson, Marston, & Erickson, 1986) have provided the limited math technical adequacy data subsequent to the IRLD research. In the Skiba et al. (1986) study, the performance of elementary students on math probes composed of addition, subtraction, multiplication, and division problems specific to grade-level curricula was examined. Probes were scored for number of correct digits written (White & Haring, 1980). Results from the Skiba et al. (1986) study are presented in Table 2.7.

In contrast to the validity studies in reading, spelling, and written expression, relations with the two criterion measures are lower. In general, the magnitude of the validity coefficients increases with the age of the subjects. Few correlations exceed .60, and the median correlation is .425 with MAT Problem-Solving and .54 with MAT Math Operations. Skiba et al. (1986) proposed two hypotheses to account for these lower than expected findings. First, there is a general concern regarding the suitability of published math tests as a criterion measure because of the limited content validity of many math tests (Freeman et al., 1983). Second, Skiba et al. (1986) demonstrated that the coefficients obtained in their study were improved significantly when each student's reading skills were included in a prediction equation. Thus, they surmised that the criterion math test also could be measuring more than just math computation skills. More research is needed in addressing this topic.

Construct validity for CBM math measures has been demonstrated in the Shinn and Marston study (1985) presented earlier. Basic multiplication and division probes differentiated students in regular education, Chapter I, and mildly handicapped programs.

TABLE 2.7. Summary of Validity Studies for Curriculum-Based Measures of Math

Study	Subjects	Criterion measure	Results
Skiba et al., 1986	185 regular education students, grades 1 to 6	MAT Operations	.54
(grade-level probes)		MAT Problem Solving	.42
(third-grade level probe)		MAT Operations	.54
		MAT Problem Solving	.43
Skiba et al., 1986	60 regular education students, grades 1 and 2	MAT Problem Solving	.26
(grade-level probes)		District CRT Basic Math Concepts	.27
(third-grade level probe)		MAT Problem Solving	.34
		District CRT Basic Math Concepts	.31
Skiba et al., 1986	65 regular education students, grades 3 and 4	MAT Problem Solving	.37
(grade-level probes)		District CRT Basic Math Concepts	.29
(third-grade level probe)		MAT Problem Solving	.45
		District CRT Basic Math Concepts	.37
Skiba et al., 1986	58 regular education students, grades 5 and 6	MAT Problem Solving	.52
(grade-level probes)		District CRT Basic Math Concepts	.67
(third-grade level probe)		MAT Problem Solving	.65
		District CRT Basic Math Concepts	.58

Additionally, mixed-operations grade-level probes distinguished the three groups at grades 5 and 6; mildly handicapped students were differentiated from regular education students in fourth grade.

Math Reliability

The CBM math reliability studies have been coordinated by Tindal (Tindal, Germann, et al., 1983; Tindal, Marston, & Deno, 1983). Results are presented in Table 2.8.

Single administrations of CBM math probes have been demonstrated to be reliable when the test–retest and parallel form estimates are examined. Interscorer agreement is high. Research is needed to determine if the aggregation of multiple math probes significantly improves the reliability of the measures, however.

At the Implementation Level/Social Policy Level

Measurement and Cost of Assessment in Time and Expense

In the traditional educational decision-making approach, school psychologists spend large amounts of time testing referred students for purposes of determining their eligibility for special education. In CBM decision-making models, special education teachers conduct most, if not all, of the testing from screening to periodic and annual reviews. However, this increased teacher-directed testing does not increase their total assessment time for two reasons. First, they no longer administer published achievement tests (e.g., WRAT, PIAT, Woodcock–Johnson) that consume part of their testing time. As a result, their time is available for the more frequent CBM assessment activities. Second, because one of the original selection criteria was time efficiency, the actual time cost of each assessment is brief. Fuchs, Wesson, Tindal, Mirkin, and Deno, (1981) observed that trained teachers average less than 2 minutes to administer, score, and graph each 1-minute reading passage. Trained teachers take about 3 minutes to administer, score, and graph each 2-minute spelling task.

With the increased responsibilities of assessment placed on special education teachers, psychologists engage in activities more commensurate with their training and often-stated preferences, such as consultation, direct interventions, teacher training, and specialized assessments. Canter's (1986) study of time spent by

TABLE 2.8. Summary of Reliability Studies of Curriculum-Based Math Measures by Domain

Study	Subjects	Type of reliability	Mixed	Add	Sub.	Mult.	Div.
Fuchs, Fuchs, & Hamlett (1988)	46 LD, 2 EMR, 14 SED students, grades 3–9	Internal consistency: Cronbach's *alpha*	.93	—	—	—	—
		Interscorer agreement on 30% of protocols	.98	—	—	—	—
Tindal, Germann, et al., 1983	30 regular education 5th graders	Test–retest (1 week)	.93	.87	.89	.79	.78
Tindal, Germann, et al., 1983	30 regular education 4th graders	2 parallel forms at same time	—	.72	.70	.61	.48
Tindal, Marston, et al., 1983	76 regular education 4th and 5th graders	Interscorer agreement	.93	.98	.99	.90	.95

psychologists from a large metropolitan school district on a variety of activities before CBM implementation in 1981 and after implementation in 1986 demonstrates an interesting finding with respect to this last issue. In the area of testing, the time spent in assessment by school psychologists is virtually identical in 1981 and 1986, about 35%. However, school psychologists tested fewer students in 1986. Canter concluded that psychologists reduced unnecessary testing and spent more time on those pupils who required comprehensive assessment. In addition to the time savings in assessment and the reallocation of roles between special educators and school psychologists, more direct cost saving is witnessed in the expenditures for assessment materials because CBM does not require the procurement of test materials (Deno, 1985).

Repeated Measurement

Another important principle embedded in CBM models is the concept of repeated measurement. Whereas traditional tests can be administered only once or perhaps twice a year, CBM procedures are designed for frequent administration (Jenkins et al., 1979). The repeated-measurement paradigm resolves several problems inherent in traditional decision making. First, repeated measurement allows the examiner to view the pupil's performance across several days at any stage in the decision-making process (e.g., problem identification, progress monitoring) in contrast to decision making based on data from only one assessment situation. In the latter instance, conditions that might have led to less than optimal performance (e.g., motivation, fatigue, unfamiliarity of the examiner) remain constant for the duration of the test session.

An example of repeated measurement is shown in Figure 2.1. In this figure, Tania's progress towards her IEP objective is monitored by having her read aloud for 1 minute two to three times per week. These procedures are maintained through the academic year, and Tania's teacher has approximately 70 to 100 solid minutes of observable, comparable reading performances with which to evaluate her progress and assay the effectiveness of the teaching program.

The advantage of repeated CBM procedures is clear in comparison to published reading tests that, at best, may provide an hour of indirect measurement of reading when testing is conducted only twice a year. The amount of systematic and direct observation of

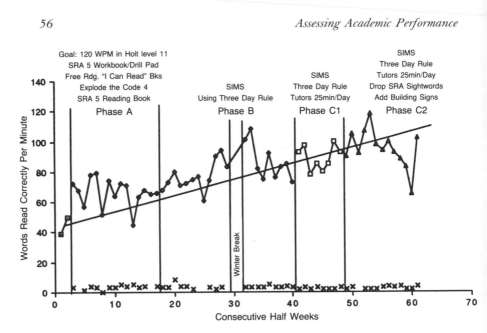

FIGURE 2-1. Tania's words correct and errors using curriculum-based measures and IEP goal line to evaluate four different modifications of her instructional program.

her reading would be far less than this figure. The repeated-measurement approach allows continual opportunity to view the pupil's progress under standardized conditions.

Time Series Analysis

Another critical component of CBM models is the time series analysis of the data. Time series analysis is the examination of the functional relationship between the data and the instructional interventions implemented by the educator over the course of time. The primary unit of analysis of effect is slope, an index of the pupil's rate of improvement, though other variables (e.g., variability, changes in level) play an important role in evaluating outcomes (see Chapter 7 for more detail). For example, in Figure 2.1, Tania was measured two or three times per week over the course of an academic year. After a period of time when her reading skills were measured in the regular education classroom without special education intervention (baseline), Tania was instructed with Science Research Associates (SRA) materials for approximately 8 weeks (Phase A). As can be seen by the slope line drawn through these data, her reading skills did not improve with this intervention. However, in Phase B, when instruction was changed to the Systematic Instructional Management System (SIMS), Tania's slope line indicated she improved considerably.

Time series analysis allows the educator to examine the pupil's progress and evaluate the effectiveness of the instructional intervention at any point during the year. The benefit of this approach is that it allows for timely decision making; Tania need not wait several months or a year to be provided with an effective instructional program designed to meet her learning needs that will help her to become a better reader. It should also be noted that the conclusion to be drawn from this example is not that SIMS is better than SRA for any particular student but that for Tania, SIMS proved a more effective instructional curriculum than SRA. With this emphasis on individual evaluation, the CBM models effectively satisfy the requirements of PL 94-142, the individualization of instruction to meet the unique needs of the learner.

Use of Local Norms in Decision Making

Deno (1985, 1986) describes the contributions of local norms to decision making as a defining characteristic of CBM. As described conceptually by Deno in Chapter 1, local norms provide an index of the expectations of the regular education environment. Although the concept of local norms is quite old, they have recently received more attention. Anastasi (1988), for example, suggests that the approach of standardizing a test on a more narrowly defined population is a "more realistic one" than use of potentially nonequivalent norms. Further, she states "local norms are more appropriate than broad national norms for many testing purposes such as . . . comparison of a child's relative achievement in different subjects or the measurement of an individual's progress over time" (p. 98).

Because of their ease of administration and time efficiency, local norms are easy to establish using curriculum-based measures. Local norms can be used to facilitate special education decisions including screening, eligibility, writing IEP objectives, monitoring progress, periodic and annual reviews, and program evaluations.

Discriminant Validity Studies Allow Reliable Differentiation of Students

It is conceivable that school decision-making practices based on traditional assessments can be characterized as unsystematic, unreliable, and, as is often implied, chaotic. In contrast, it has been argued that the social policy of eligibility decision making regarding mild handicaps is, indeed, quite orderly. This argument is premised on the hypothesis that researchers have investigated the wrong variables (i.e., performance on published, norm-referenced measures of intelligence and achievement) with respect to the criterion of certification of students as handicapped. For Shinn et al. (1987), order in decision making is evidenced by specifically examining the level of achievement within the regular education curriculum for students who are certified as handicapped.

After reviewing all the available CBM investigations that attempted to ascertain the degree to which CBM measures could differentiate different groups of students (i.e., learning disabled, Chapter I, low-achieving, and regular-education students), Shinn et al. (1988) concluded that CBM procedures reliably differentiated the students into unique groups. Students placed into programs for learning disabilities via extensive traditional assessment procedures earned extremely low scores on CBM achievement measures compared to their peers in the regular education classroom.

In the Shinn et al. (1987) study, for example, the performances of 638 students in grades 1 to 6 who had been placed in LD programs were compared with a random sample of students who were (1) receiving remedial Chapter I services and (2) who were receiving no supplemental programming as part of their regular education. All the LD students had an IEP objective in reading and had been placed within the context of a criterion of significant ability–achievement discrepancies. Students in the three groups were compared on CBM reading measures and were reliably differentiated. Whereas the shapes of distributions of all three groups relative to each other were similar across grades, there was little overlap between and among groups. For example in fifth grade, 75% of the LD students performed below the lower quartile of Chapter I students. Similarly, 75% of Chapter I students performed below the lower quartile of regular-education-only students. Consistently, the median performance of LD students was below the fifth percentile of the reading achievement of regular education students, and three out of four LD students earned scores below the 10th percentile of the local normative group.

To summarize the results of the four studies that used CBM to differentiate intact groups (Deno et al., 1983; Shinn & Marston, 1985; Shinn et al., 1986, 1987), M. R. Shinn (unpublished data) converted the mean differences in reading performance among the three groups into effect sizes. Effect sizes were determined by subtracting the mean of the learning-disabled sample from either (1) the mean of low-achieving groups and/or (2) the mean of the regular-education-only groups and dividing by the standard deviation of the respective group. For the primary grades (i.e., 1 to 3), the median effect size between learning-disabled students and low achievers was −.69. Between learning-disabled students and regular-education-only students, the median effect size was −1.74. For the intermediate grades (i.e., 4 through 6), the median effect sizes between learning-disabled students and low achievers and regular-education students were −1.15 and −2.18, respectively.

Continuity across Special Education Decisions

In CBM, the discontinuity problem of traditional testing is resolved by using a common standard for decision making, the regular education curricula. Regardless of what decision is to be made, the same basic measurement strategies (i.e., simple, repeated measures of performance within curricula) are used in the decision-making process. What changes across decisions is the level of the curriculum used in decision making and the criterion standard. The continuity of decision making within a CBM decision-making model used in Minneapolis Public Schools (Marston & Magnusson, 1985, 1988) is presented in Table 2.9. The area of reading is used as the curriculum example.

School districts often use CBM procedures to make special education screening decisions. The goal of the process is to determine if a referred student is sufficiently different from regular education peers that further assessment is warranted. As shown in Table 2.9, reading samples from grade-level materials are collected and compared to local norms of grade-level peers (Marston & Magnusson, 1985).

When decisions are made regarding a student's eligibility for mildly handicapped services, the choice of materials and decision-making standards require a student to be tested on curriculum materials *below* their current grade placement. The scores that are obtained are compared to students at lower grades as well. This process is entitled survey level assessment (Marston & Magnusson, 1985). In addition to assisting in determining special education eligibility, interpretation of CBM survey level assessment data also identifies student curricular skills that need further testing. One of the difficulties that plague many criterion-referenced tests is that

TABLE 2.9. A Sample of the Continuity of CBM Assessment across the Special Education Decisions in the Area of Reading

Special education decision	CBM material	Comparison standard
Screening	Typical grade-level basal reader	Grade-level peers
Eligibility	Basal readers from lower grade levels	Students at lower grade levels
IEP planning	Basal readers from lower grade levels	Norms from grade-level peers
		Norms from lower-grade peers
		Instructional placement criteria
		Expected rates of progress
		Mastery criteria
Monitoring instructional progress	Basal reader from IEP objective material	Criterion derived from IEP planning
Periodic and annual review/exit	Average grade-level basal reader	Grade-level peers
		Comparisons of progress in regular versus special education

teachers often do not know which parts of the test to give. As a result, entire criterion-referenced batteries are administered at a considerable cost in time or are not utilized at all. Because of its general testing nature, survey level testing samples many types of skills in a content area in a short period of time. By a careful process of error analysis of student performance and by familiarizing themselves with the curricular demands at a given grade, teachers may conduct concise assessments to document student skill areas that need a more thorough assessment. For example, Dave is a third grader with many spelling problems. Survey level assessment began by comparing Dave's spelling performance on second- and first-grade spelling words to the appropriate grade standard. As a result, it was determined that Dave spells much as first graders do on the first-grade spelling words. During the Survey level assessment, it was observed that he misspelled several words with the pattern CVC-e (consonant-vowel-consonant-silent "e") such as "bone" and "home." With a knowledge of the curricular demands, assessors then can follow up these results with more detailed assessment and analysis of skill components.

As evidenced in Table 2.9, instructional planning within CBM is constrained mostly to the writing of IEP objectives that are based on student performance data within the curriculum. Each IEP objective is individualized by varying the level of curriculum measurement material and the criterion for success. Reading data obtained from different levels of the local curriculum are used to determine goal material. In the case of the seventh grader who reads fourth-grade material like a fourth grader, the multi-disciplinary team may expect the student to read fifth-grade material like a typical fifth grader in 1 year. Among the methods for selecting the success criterion for the IEP objective, a number are developed through the use of local norms (see Chapter 5 for more detail).

Progress monitoring represents another decision area in which CBM can be used. Within the CBM framework, school personnel continuously monitor the effectiveness of their instructional interventions and student progress toward IEP goals that have been written. The curriculum material specified in the IEP objective constitutes the material to be used to monitor progress. In many districts using CBM, special education students are assessed on a regular basis, usually once or twice per week, on CBM measures from the IEP objective domain (Germann & Tindal, 1985; Marston & Magnusson, 1985). The student's rate of progress is compared to the expected rate of progress designed to meet the normative criterion. Successful instructional programs are those that result in progress equal to or greater than the expected rate. Unsuccessful instructional programs, those not resulting in the expected rate of growth, are changed.

Tied to monitoring of progress towards IEP objectives is a systematic periodic and annual review process. These decision-making activities are systematic comparisons of the relative standing of special education students with respect to local normative performance of grade-level peers in the special education students' grade-level curricula. At the times in which local norm data are collected, special education students are retested on CBM materials and compared to the local norms. For example, the special education student may perform at the second percentile at the beginning of the year and by midyear and year's end perform at the 12th and 17th percentiles, respectively. Students who are making significant progress are reducing the skill discrepancy between themselves and peers. Students who are falling further behind have their instructional programs reevaluated. When these results are combined with data corresponding to progress towards the IEP objective, a robust picture is obtained of special education effectiveness. Students who are attaining their IEP objective but falling further behind their peers may need to have their IEP objectives changed. Data derived from these periodic reviews also can be used to consider termination of services or reduction in level of service. Students who have made significant progress towards IEP objectives and/or reduced peer discrepancies may be placed in a less restrictive environment.

An alternative approach to program evaluation, based on CBM procedures, is time-series analysis of the effectiveness of general education delivery systems. Marston (1988) examined the reading growth of mildly handicapped students placed only in regular education versus placement in resource classrooms. He concluded that the slope of reading improvement was significantly greater when students were instructed in special education compared to regular education.

Differences between CBA Models

The term curriculum-based assessment has become popular in recent years (Tucker, 1985). It is important to note that in addition to the fluency-based model of CBM, there is more than one approach to curriculum-based assessment, including *accuracy-based models* (Gickling & Havertape, 1981; Gickling & Thompson, 1985; Hargis, 1987) and *criterion-referenced models* (Blankenship, 1985; Idol, Nevin, & Paolucci-Whitcomb, 1986). Broadly defined, curriculum-based assessment (CBA) is any set of measurement procedures that use "direct observation and recording of a student's performance in the local curriculum as a basis for gathering information to make instructional decisions" (Deno, 1987). In a brief review of the different CBA models for the California Association of School Psychologists Newsletter, Frisby (1987) identified four common principles:

1. The measurement procedures are direct. Students are assessed directly in materials that they are being instructed from in the classroom.
2. Test administration is of short duration. Measures are administered typically in 1 to 3 minutes for each identified academic behavior.
3. The design of the procedures allows for frequent and repeat-

ed measurement. Data can be collected one to five times weekly.
4. The procedures are "experimental." The data are graphed and charted systematically to allow for monitoring of student progress.

In practice, however, the different CBA models differ in these principles to varying degrees. Further, accuracy-based and criterion-referenced CBA models differ from CBM in a number of other dimensions, including (1) primary purpose of the measurement, (2) the academic behavior that is measured, (3) the type(s) of student responses, (4) approach to planning effective instructional interventions, (5) the level of focus of measurement material for monitoring progress, (6) standardized measurement materials and testing formats, (7) availability of technical adequacy, and (8) utility for making other educational decisions besides instructional planning and student progress monitoring.

Accuracy-Based CBA Model

Gickling and his associates (Gickling & Havertape, 1981; Gickling & Thompson, 1985; Hargis, 1987) pioneered the current movement of tying assessment directly to curricula. The major outcome measure for Gickling and his associates is an expression of per centage of correct student responses. Therefore, this model is best conceptualized as an accuracy model. The major use of CBA is for instructional planning purposes. As stated by Gickling and Thompson (1985), CBA "provides teachers with the specificity to pinpoint where to begin instructional sequences." Its specific purpose is to "eliminate the instructional mismatch between the skills of low-achieving and mainstreamed students and the inordinate demands placed upon them by their curriculum assignments. . . ."

Frisby (1987) typifies the Gickling et al. model as task analytic in nature. He describes the model as placing exclusive assessment emphasis on an analysis of the task demands of instructional materials that students are to learn. In practice, assessment is linked directly to the instructional process. Assessment of subtask performance is part of the actual instructional process. Teachers are encouraged, if not expected, to develop their own instructional materials (Hargis, 1987) based on assessment results. Thus, Gickling's model of CBA might be viewed more as an intervention model rather than an assessment model *per se*.

According to Tindal (1988), the accuracy-based CBA model uses primarily production-type responses to measure student performance. For example, students read aloud passages 100 to 150 words in length. This basic datum is converted to a ratio of the percentage of "knowns" (corrects) to "unknowns" (errors). However, examination of two sources of CBA materials (Gickling & Havertape, 1981; Hargis, 1987) provides instances in which selection-type responses (e.g., draw a line under) are used. The academic focus centers mostly on reading and math (Tindal, 1988). After instructional placement of the student is established using the known-to-unknown ratio, the measurement focus changes to the evaluation of academic learning time, the amount of time a student spends in relevant content that he/she can perform with high success (Denham & Lieberman, 1980).

With respect to its approach to instructional planning, the accuracy-based model is deductive in its approach. That is, it presumes that with knowledge of assessment results effective instructional programs will be implemented. Gickling and Thompson (1985) refer to CBA as another type of "diagnostic prescriptive process." Once correct instructional placement has been determined via CBA assessment, student progress is assured. This presumption is established further by Hargis (1987), who argues that the "result of a good match between instructional material and student is a high level of performance" (p. 13).

As pointed out earlier, in the Gickling model, student progress is assessed indirectly using academic learning time (ALT). For example, during reading instruction, ALT is measured and graphed. Gickling and Thompson (1985) maintain that the emergence of the ALT concept has provided a strong alternative to the traditional practices of measuring students' progress. Among the benefits of using ALT to monitor student progress, Gickling and Havertape (1981) consider (1) the specific information relevant for instruction and (2) sensitivity to improvement as the most salient. Increases in ALT are used to validate effective instructional programs. Examples of use of ALT as an indicator of effective instructional programs have been offered (Gickling & Thompson, 1985). Although there is a correlation between reading achievement and ALT, it is not necessarily a direct measure of reading.

To date, little evidence for technical adequacy for the accuracy-based measures has been offered, other than their content validity. In part, this lack of data results from the authors' lack of standardized procedures. As Gickling and Havertape (1981) state, "We prefer the data be collected and recorded systematically but do not have a preference about how this is to be done" (p. 21).

Finally, little explicit use for other special education decisions besides instructional planning and student progress monitoring has been identified. Although Gickling and Havertape (1981) conceptualize assessment as composed of four phases (i.e., screening, identification, instructional planning, and measurement of progress), they prescribe procedures only for instructionally planning. One could infer that screening and eligibility decisions would be made when failed instructional programs, those designed and evaluated using CBA measures, are documented.

Criterion-Referenced Models

The criterion-referenced model(s) of CBA is exemplified by the work of Blankenship (1985) and Idol (Idol-Maestas, 1983). In this model, CBA is defined as ". . . the practice of obtaining direct and frequent measures of a student's performance on a series of sequentially arranged objectives from the curriculum used in the classroom" (Blankenship & Lilly, 1981, p. 81). Similar to Gickling's accuracy-based model (Gickling & Havertape, 1981), the primary purpose of administering CBAs is to provide teachers with information for instructional planning (Idol et al., 1986). In an analogous manner to Gickling and his colleagues, this model of CBA may be viewed best as a teaching model rather than a testing one. As Blankenship (1985) states, "The essence of the approach is the linking of assessment to curriculum and instruction."

Assessment proceeds through a process in which the skills to be taught from the curriculum are listed and an objective for each is written. Specific curricular items are selected and combined to make a test. An acceptable performance criterion is established, and students are tested for mastery of each objective (Blankenship, 1985). Examples of CBAs have been provided in the domains of math, reading, spelling, science, dictionary skills, direction following, and use of study skills (Idol et al., 1986).

The suggested assessment measures and type of data collected vary widely according to the specific instructional objectives taken from the different academic areas. In reading, for example, data on multiple measures are collected. Based on sample passages taken from the student's reading curriculum, the percentage of words read accurately and comprehension questions answered correctly, as well as the number of words read per minute, are calculated (Idol et al., 1986). Additional measurement of student performance may be collected on behaviors such as number of minutes required to complete a silent reading assignment and number of workbook pages and homework assignments completed at a specific performance level (Idol-Maestas, 1983). In contrast to the other CBA models, the criterion-referenced model can be employed in more than the basic skill areas. Both Idol and Blankenship maintain that CBA can used with any type of curriculum material.

The criterion-referenced CBA model relies primarily on production-type responses to assess student performance. The types of responses are broader than those of the fluency-based and accuracy-based models and include behaviors such as (1) providing written answers to math word problems, (2) writing dictated spelling words, and (3) numbering words in alphabetical order (Blankenship, 1985; Idol et al., 1986). Selection-type responses are also evident in some CBAs. For example, in assessing the student's dictionary skill, students are required to cross out words that would not be found on a dictionary page (Idol et al., 1986). Additionally, less-well-defined behaviors, such as "the student will read and discuss" or "describe and illustrate," are suggested (Idol et al., 1986).

This CBA model is designed primarily for continuous assessment of short-term instructional objectives. Frequent measurement of a student's performance takes place on a set(s) of current instructional objectives over time. For example, after receiving instruction, students are administered a test developed to sample the lesson's objectives to assess their mastery of the skills taught. Less attention is given to long-term monitoring of student progress, although Blankenship (1985) proposes that long-term retention can be assessed by the periodic readministration of the CBA throughout the year. To accomplish long-term monitoring, however, Idol et al., (1986) suggest that multiple forms of the CBA for each objective must be constructed.

Typically, test administration within the criterion-referenced CBA model(s) is less than standardized. As a case in point, the frequency with which the CBAs should be administered and the specific procedures for monitoring a student's performance are not explained. Rather, the authors present a series of test item examples that teachers can use to guide their own development of test items (Blankenship, 1985; Idol et al., 1986). Standardized instructions for administration of each objective's tests are noticeably absent.

To date, information on technical adequacy for the criterion-referenced measures is absent from the literature. As with the accuracy-based CBA model, the lack of research on the measurement procedures proposed in this model may partly result from the lack of specified standardized procedures.

Evidence for the use of the CBA procedures presented in this model for decisions other than instructional plan cannot be found. Although Blankenship (1985) states that the data collected from the administration of CBAs can provide the basis for decisions regarding referrals, IEP planning, and determining the least restrictive environment, systematic procedures for making these decisions are not detailed.

Summary

Although both accuracy- and criterion-referenced models of CBA and CBM generally use student performance in the curriculum as the basic decision-making standard, the models differ on a number of salient dimensions that are not necessarily incompatible if the school psychologist discriminates which special education decision is being made. A summary comparison of both accuracy- and criterion-referenced based models of CBA with CBM is presented in Table 2.10.

Implementation of CBM and the Changing Role of the School Psychologist

Keogh (1972) observed that school psychologists limit their diagnostic contribution to the educational process when they assume a role primarily as a test examiner. She argued that "a somewhat different model of school psychology be adopted if services to exceptional children are to be effective." Reschly (1987) concluded that the conventional testing model is inadequate, stating "The amount of time and energy now devoted to preplacement and reevaluations [in special education], which are dominated by determination of eligibility, represents excessively costly and ineffective use of resources." Reynolds (1982), who agrees that there is a need for change in school psychology, argues that the need arises because education is changing.

TABLE 2.10. A Comparison of CBM, Accuracy-Based, and Criterion-Referenced (CR) Models of CBA

Comparison point	CBM	Accuracy-based	CR
Primary purpose of assessment	Direct measurement of student progress	Instructional placement	Instructional content
What is measured	Fluency	Accuracy	Varies
Type of student response	Production	Production/ALT	Varies
Approach to instructional planning	Inductive	Deductive	Deductive
Focus of material for monitoring progress	Long term	Indirect measurement (ALT)	Short term
Standardized measurement materials and test formats	Yes	No	No
Data on technical adequacy	Yes	No	No
Evidence for use for other decisions	Screening, eligibility, program evaluation	Indirect measure of student progress	No

. . . public education has changed: student bodies have become more heterogeneous, new structures have begun to appear, and new functions and roles are demanded of teachers, building principals, school psychologists, and other specialists. Most of the changes derive from the mandated provision of services to populations that, heretofore, were considered marginal, that is, the handicapped, minority, economically disadvantaged, bilingual, migrant, and other children and youth who have been systematically set aside or excluded from the mainstreams of society and the schools. (p. 104)

This state of affairs has obvious implications for the role of the school psychologist and necessitates ". . . an in-depth analysis of the emerging rights of children and the new principles being applied to the education of 'marginal' children" (Reynolds, 1982). To make the transition, Reynolds (1982) has identified nine clusters of competency school psychologists must possess to make a successful change: (1) consultation, (2) individualized assessment, (3) diverse social structures, (4) individualized instruction, (5) deliberate psychological education, (6) parent involvement, (7) teaching basic skills, (8) group management, and (9) the law and judicial procedures. Whereas all clusters are essential for improving services for handicapped students, it is the individualized assessment of "marginal children" that fits into the CBM perspective. Reynolds (1982) differentiates individualized assessment from traditional assessment in four important ways. First, he emphasizes the significance of directing assessment toward the instructional needs of the child, stating that "the assessments should help to design appropriate instructional programs for students." Second, he argued that "assessments should be mainly curriculum-based or behavioral" so that they relate to a student's instructional and behavioral context. Third, he maintained that assessments should be direct, "based heavily on direct observations rather than on presumed predispositional or underlying traits." Finally, he stipulated that assessment must be sensitive to the student's growth and that they be "highly specific to the domains of instruction and so designed that individuals have clear opportunities to become aware of their own progress. . . ."

Obviously, these remarks are congruent with the purposes of CBM implementation. It is oriented to instruction, is data driven, relates to the curriculum, and is behaviorally based. As school psychologists move away from the "gatekeeper" status to consultation and direct service, the CBM model will help guide their decision making on pupil progress and intervention effectiveness. It is our belief that as the role of the school psychologist changes attraction to CBM models will increase.

More Prereferral Intervention

When assessment becomes more teacher directed, school psychologists may engage in more prereferral interventions and work to modify the mainstream regular education classroom (Trachtman, 1981). At a demonstration school in the Minneapolis Public Schools, for example, students considered for referral are not referred for eligibility determination. Rather, the classroom performance of the student(s) that the teacher is concerned about is monitored on a frequent basis, and at least two different regular education interventions are tried with the student. If the pupil does not respond to these interventions as evidenced by the achievement data, a referral to the special education program may be initiated. This type of model provides school psychologists with unique opportunities for instructional and/or behavioral consultation: they can adopt a problem-solving approach to a psychological services as opposed to psychometric approach. Further, they do not have to wait for actual referral to begin work with a student. Thus, the continuous monitoring of a "high-risk" child provides an opportunity for the psychologist to move directly into a consulting situation with the regular education teacher.

Instructional and Behavioral Consultant

The school psychology professional literature is replete with numerous calls for the provision of more indirect and direct services to children, teachers, and parents (Sewell, 1981). Importantly, this literature does not distinguish between the services delivered to special education or regular education students. Further, some school psychologists argue that school psychological services should not end when eligibility is determined but should become more intensified at the point of certification as handicapped (Reschly, 1982; Shinn, 1986). As described earlier in this chapter, when the impact of a change in assessment models to one based on CBM, some impact on the practices of school psychologists in the district has been demonstrated. Canter (1986) demonstrated a significant increase in indirect services. Similarly, school psychologists significantly increased their time providing direct services from 1.5% in 1981 to 6% in 1986, a 400% increase.

The trend towards more psychological service delivery is viewed as a significant improvement by psychologists who have stated for more than 20 years that they prefer to spend more time in consultation and treatment activities. Utilization of CBM, which provides a common metric across the psychoeducational decision areas, promotes the idea that school psychologists can engage in more than "gatekeeping" activities. Because CBM procedures are linked directly to program planning, the school psychologist may take an active role in planning instruction, setting goals, and writing IEP objectives. Further, because CBM procedures are sensitive to pupil growth, they allow the school psychologist to play an instrumental role in determining pupil progress and making decisions about treatment and intervention effectiveness. This role may facilitate further the role of the school psychologist in participating in alternative intervention planning and implementation. Finally, the "common metric" of CBM facilitates the task of program evaluation, a function that seems consonant with the delivery of effective school psychological services. Indeed, it would appear that movement of assessment activities into the areas of program planning, progress monitoring, and program evaluation would promise increments of the consultation and treatment activities of the school psychologist.

ACKNOWLEDGMENTS

I wish to thank Nancy M. Knutson for her contributions to the CBA models section of this chapter and Vicki L. Collins, Nancy M. Knutson, and W. David Tilly III for their efforts in compiling the CBM reliability and validity tables. They all are doctoral students in school psychology at the University of Oregon.

REFERENCES

American Psychological Association, American Educational Research Association, and National Council on Measurement in Education. (1985). *Standards for educational and psychological tests*. Washington: American Psychological Association.

Anastasi, A. (1988). *Psychological testing* (6th ed.). New York: Macmillan.

Beery, K. E. & Buktenica, N. (1967). *Developmental test of visual–motor integration*. Chicago: Follett.

Berk, R. (1984). *Screening and diagnosis of children with learning disabilities*. Springfield, IL: Charles C. Thomas.

Blankenship, C. (1985). Using curriculum-based assessment data to make instructional decisions. *Exceptional Children, 52*, 233–238.

Blankenship, C., & Lilly, S. (1981). *Mainstreaming students with learning and behavior problems: Techniques for the classroom teacher*. New York: Holt, Rinehart & Winston.

Boyan, C. (1985). California's new eligibility criteria: Legal and program implications. *Exceptional Children, 52*, 131–141.

Canter, A. (1986). *1986 time/task study*. Minneapolis: Minneapolis Public Schools, Department of Special Education, Psychological Services.

Carver, R. P. (1974). Two dimensions of tests: Psychometric and edumetric. *American Psychologist, 29*, 512–518.

Commission on Reading. (1985). *Becoming a nation of readers: The report of the commission on reading*. Washington: The National Institute of Education.

Cronbach, L. J., & Furby, L. (1970). How we should measure "change"—or should we? *Psychological Bulletin, 1*, 68–80.

Denham, C., & Lieberman, A. (Eds.). (1980). *Time to learn*. Washington: US Department of Education, National Institute of Education.

Deno, S. L. (1985). Curriculum-based measurement: The emerging alternative. *Exceptional Children, 52,* 219–232.

Deno, S. L. (1986). Formative evaluation of individual programs: A new role for school psychologists. *School Psychology Review, 15,* 358–374.

Deno, S. L. (1987). Curriculum-based measurement. *Teaching Exceptional Children, 20,* 41.

Deno, S. L., Marston, D., & Mirkin, P. K. (1982). Valid measurement procedures for continuous evaluation of written expression. *Exceptional Children, 48,* 368–371.

Deno, S. L., Marston, D., Mirkin, P. K., Lowry, L., Sindelar, P., & Jenkins, J. (1982). *The use of standard tasks to measure achievement in reading, spelling, and written expression: A normative and developmental study* (Research Report No. 87). Minneapolis: University of Minnesota Institute for Research on Learning Disabilities (ERIC Document Reproduction Service No. ED 227 129).

Deno, S. L., Marston, D., Shinn, M. R., & Tindal, G. (1983). Oral reading fluency: A simple datum for scaling reading disability. *Topics in Learning and Learning Disability, 2,* 53–59.

Deno, S. L., Mirkin, P. K., & Chiang, B. (1982). Identifying valid measures of reading. *Exceptional Children, 49,* 36–45.

Deno, S. L., Mirkin, P. K., Lowry, L., & Kuehnle, K. (1980). *Relationships among simple measures of spelling and performance on standardized achievement tests* (Research Report No. 21). Minneapolis: Institute for Research on Learning Disabilities, University of Minnesota.

Deno, S. L., Mirkin, P. K., & Marston, D. (1980). *Relationships among simple measures of written expression and performance on standardized achievement tests* (Research Report No. 22). Minneapolis: University of Minnesota Institute for Research on Learning Disabilities.

Diana v. St. Board of Education, CA No. C-70-37 (N. D. Cal., July 1970) (consent decree).

Dunn, L., & Markwardt, F. (1970). *Peabody individual achievement test.* Circle Pines, MN: American Guidance Service.

Durost, W. N., Bixler, H. H., Wrightstone, J. W., Prescott, G. A., & Balow, I. H. (1971). *Metropolitan Achievement Test.* New York: Harcourt, Brace, & Jovanovich.

Eaton, M., & Lovitt, T. C. (1972). Achievement tests versus direct and daily measurement. In G. Semb (Ed.), *Behavior analysis in education.* Lawrence, KS: University of Kansas.

Epps, S., Ysseldyke, J. E., & McGue, M. (1984). "I know one when I see one"—Differentiating LD and non-LD students. *Learning Disability Quarterly, 7,* 89–101.

Forness, S. R., & Kavale, K. A. (1987). De-psychologizing special education, In R. B. Rutherford, C. M. Nelson, & S. R. Forness (Eds.), *Severe behavior disorders of children and youth* (pp. 2–14). Boston: College Hill Press.

Freeman, D. J., Kuhs, T. M., Porter, A. C., Floden, R. E., Schmidt, W. H., & Schwille, J. R. (1983). Do textbooks and tests define a national curriculum in elementary school mathematics? *Elementary School Journal, 83,* 501–513.

Frisby, C. (1987). Alternative assessment committee report: Curriculum-based assessment. *CASP Today, 36,* 15–26.

Fuchs, D., Fuchs, L. S., Benowitz, S., & Berringer, K. (1987). Norm-referenced tests: Are they valid for use with handicapped students? *Exceptional Children, 54,* 263–271.

Fuchs, L. S., & Deno, S. L. (1981). *The relationship between curriculum-based mastery measures and standardized achievement tests in reading* (Research Report No. 57). Minneapolis: University of Minnesota Institute for Research on Learning Disabilities (ERIC Document Reproduction Service No. ED 212 662).

Fuchs, L. S., Deno, S. L., & Marston, D. (1983). Improving the reliability of curriculum-based measures of academic skills for psychoeducational decision making. *Diagnostique, 8,* 135–149.

Fuchs, L. S., Fuchs, D., & Hamlett, C. L. (1988). *Computer applications to curriculum-based measurement: Effects of teacher feedback systems.* Unpublished manuscript, Peabody College, Vanderbilt University, Nashville, TN.

Fuchs, L. S., Fuchs, D., & Maxwell, S. (1988). The validity of informal reading comprehension measures. *Remedial and Special Education, 9*(2), 20–28.

Fuchs, L. S, Fuchs, D., & Warren, L. (1982). *Special education practice in evaluating student progress towards goals* (Research Report No. 82). Minneapolis: University of Minnesota Institute for Research on Learning Disabilities (ERIC Document Reproduction Service No. ED 224 197).

Fuchs, L. S., Tindal, G., & Deno, S. L. (1984). *Methodological issues in curriculum based reading assessment. Diagnostique, 9,* 191–207.

Fuchs, L. S, Tindal, G., Fuchs, D., Shinn, M. R., Deno, S. L., & Germann, G. (1983). *Technical adequacy of basal readers' mastery tests: Holt basic series* (Research Report No. 130). Minneapolis: University of Minnesota Institute for Research on Learning Disabilities.

Fuchs, L. S, Tindal, G., Shinn, M. R., Fuchs, D., Deno, S. L., & Germann, G. (1983). *Technical adequacy of basal readers' mastery tests: Ginn 720 series* (Research Report No. 122). Minneapolis: University of Minnesota Institute for Research on Learning Disabilities.

Galagan, J. E. (1985). Psychoeducational testing: Turn out the lights, the party's over. *Exceptional Children, 52,* 288–298.

Germann, G., & Tindal, G. (1985). An application of curriculum-based assessment: The use of direct and repeated measurement. *Exceptional Children, 52,* 244–265.

Gickling, E., & Havertape, J. (1981). *Curriculum-based assessment (CBA).* Minneapolis: National School Psychology Inservice Training Network.

Gickling, E., & Thompson, V. (1985). A personal view of curriculum-based assessment. *Exceptional Children, 52,* 205–218.

Goldwasser, E., Meyers, J., Christenson, S., & Graden, J. (1984). The impact of P. L. 94-142 on the practice of school psychology: A national survey. *Psychology in the Schools, 20,* 153–165.

Hammill, D., & Larsen, S. (1978). *Test of Written Language.* Austin, TX: Pro-Ed.

Hargis, C. H. (1987). *Curriculum-based assessment: A primer.* Springfield, IL: Charles C. Thomas.

Hively, W., & Reynolds, M. C. (Eds.). (1975). *Domain-reference testing in special education.* Reston, VA: The Council for Exceptional Children.

Hobson V. Hansen, 269 F. Supp. 401 (D. D. C. 1967). Affirmed, Smuck v. Hobson, 408 F. 2d. 175, (D. C. Cir. 1969).

Howell, K. W., & Kaplan, J. S. (1980). *Diagnosing basic skills: A handbook for deciding what to teach.* Columbus, OH: Charles Merrill.

Hughes, J. (1979). Consistency of administrators and psychologists actual and ideal perceptions of school psychologists' activities. *Psychology in the Schools, 16,* 234–239.

Hunt, K. W. (1966). Recent measures in syntactic development. *Elementary English, 42,* 732–739.

Idol, L., Nevin, A., & Paolucci-Whitcomb, P. (1986). *Models of curriculum-based assessment.* Rockville, MD: Aspen.

Idol-Maestas, L. (1983). *Special educator's consultation handbook.* Rockville, MD: Aspen.

Jastak, S. E., & Jastak, S. R. (1978). *Wide range achievement test.* Wilmington, DE: Jastak Associates.

Jenkins, J. R., Deno, S. L., & Mirkin, P. K. (1979). Measuring pupil progress toward the least restrictive environment. *Learning Disability Quarterly, 2,* 81–92.

Jenkins, J. R. & Pany, D. (1978). Standardized achievement tests: How useful for special education? *Exceptional Children, 44,* 448–453.

Karlsen, B., Madden, R., & Gardner, E. (1975). *Stanford Diagnostic Reading Test* (2nd ed.). San Antonio, TX: The Psychological Corporation.

Keogh, B. K. (1972). Psychological evaluation of exceptional children: Old hangups and new directions. *Journal of School Psychology, 10,* 141–145.

Koppitz, E. M. (1963). *The Bender gestalt test for young children.* New York: Grune and Stratton.

Larry P. v. Riles, 343 F. Suppl. 1306 (N. D. Cal. 1972) (preliminary injunction), aff'd 502 F. 2d. 963 (9th Cir. 1974); 495. Supp. 926 (N. D. Cal. 1979) (decision on merits) aff'd (9th cir. no. 80-427, Jan. 23, 1984). Order modifying judgment. C-71-2270 RFP, September 25, 1986.

Larsen, S., & Hammill, D. (1976). *Test of Written Spelling.* Austin, TX: Pro-Ed.

Lee, L., & Canter, S. (1971). Developmental sentence scoring: A clinical procedure for estimating syntactic development in children's spontaneous speech. *Journal of Speech and Hearing Disorders, 36,* 315–340.

Madden, R., Gardner, E., Rudman, H., Karlsen, B., & Merwin, J. (1978). *Stanford Achievement Test.* New York: Harcourt Brace Jovanovich.

Marston, D. (1982). *The technical adequacy of direct, repeated measurement of academic skills in low-achieving elementary students.* Unpublished doctoral dissertation, Minneapolis: University of Minnesota.

Marston, D. (1988). The effectiveness of special education: A time series analysis of reading performance in regular and special education settings. *The Journal of Special Education, 21*(4), 13–26.

Marston, D., & Deno, S. L. (1981). *The reliability of simple, direct measures of written expression* (Research Report No. 50). Minneapolis: University of Minnesota Institute for Research on Learning Disabilities.

Marston, D., & Deno, S. L. (1982). *Implementation of direct and repeated measurement in the school setting* (Research Report No. 106). Minneapolis: University of Minnesota Institute for Research on Learning Disabilities.

Marston, D., Fuchs, L. S., & Deno, S. L. (1986). Measuring pupil progress: A comparison of standardized achievement tests and curriculum-related measures. *Diagnostique, 11,* 77–90.

Marston, D., Lowry, L., Deno, S. L., & Mirkin, P. K. (1981). *An analysis of learning trends in simple measures of reading, spelling, and written expression: A longitudinal study* (Research Report No. 49). Minneapolis: University of Minnesota Institute for Research on Learning Disabilities.

Marston, D., & Magnusson, D. (1985). Implementing curriculum-based measurement in special and regular education settings. *Exceptional Children, 52,* 266–276.

Marston, D., & Magnusson, D. (1988). Curriculum-based measurement: District level implementation. In J. L. Graden, J. E. Zins, & M. J. Curtis (Eds.), *Alternative educational delivery systems. Enhancing instructional options for all students* (pp. 137–172). Kent, OH: National Association of School Psychologists.

Marston, D., Mirkin, P. K., & Deno, S. L. (1984). Curriculum-based measurement: An alternative to traditional screening, referral, and identification. *Journal of Special Education, 18,* 109–118.

Marston, D., Tindal, G., & Deno, S. L. (1983). *A comparison of standardized achievement tests and direct measurement techniques in measuring student progress* (Research Report No. 126). Minneapolis: University of Minnesota Institute for Research on Learning Disabilities.

Mirkin, P. K. (1980). Conclusions. In J. E. Ysseldyke & M. L. Thurlow (Eds.), *The special education assessment and decision-making process: Seven case studies.* Minneapolis: University of Minnesota Institute for Research on Learning Disabilities.

Mitchell, P. (1985). *The ninth mental measurements yearbook.* Highland Park, NJ: Gryphon Press.

Poland, S., Thurlow, M. L., Ysseldyke, J. E., & Mirkin, P. K. (1982). Current psychoeducational assessment and decision-making practices as reported by directors of special education. *Journal of School Psychology, 20,* 171–179.

Popham, W. J., & Baker, E. L. (1970). *Systematic instruction.* Englewood Cliffs, NJ: Prentice-Hall.

Reschly, D. (1982). Assessing mild retardation: The influence of adaptive behavior, sociocultural status and prospects for nonbiased assessment. In C. Reynolds & T. Gutkin (Eds.), *The handbook of school psychology.* New York: John Wiley & Sons.

Reschly, D. J. (1987). Learning characteristics of mildly handicapped students: Implications for classification, placement, and programming. In M. C. Reynolds, M. C. Wang, & H. J. Walberg (Eds.), *The handbook of special education: Research and practice* (Vol. 1). Oxford, England: Pergamon.

Reynolds, M. C. (1982). The rights of children: A challenge to school psychologists. In T. R. Kratochwill (Ed.), *Advances in school psychology: Vol. 2* (pp. 97–118). Hillsdale, NJ: Lawrence Erlbaum Associates.

Salvia, J., & Ysseldyke, J. E. (1982). *Assessment in special and remedial education* (2nd ed.). Boston: Houghton-Mifflin.

Salvia, J., & Ysseldyke, J. E. (1985). *Assessment in special and remedial education* (3rd ed.). Boston: Houghton-Mifflin.

Samuels, S. J. (1979). The method of repeated readings. *The Reading Teacher, 32,* 1–6.

Sandoval, J. (1987). Larry who? Coping with the extended ban on IQ tests for black children. *Trainer's Forum: The Newsletter of Trainers of School Psychologists, 7,* 2–3.

Sewell, T. (1981). Shaping the course of school psychology: Another perspective. *School Psychology Review, 11,* 232–242.

Shapiro, E. S. (1987). *Behavioral assessment in school psychology.* Hillsdale, NJ: Lawrence Erlbaum Associates.

Shapiro, E. S., & Derr, T. F. (1987). An examination of the overlap between reading curricula and standardized achievement tests. *The Journal of Special Education, 21,* 59–67.

Shinn, M. R. (1981). *A comparison of psychometric and functional differences between students labeled learning disabled and low achieving.* Unpublished doctoral dissertation, Minneapolis: University of Minnesota.

Shinn, M. R. (1986). Does anyone care what happens after the refer–test–place sequence: The systematic evaluation of special education program effectiveness. *School Psychology Review, 15,* 49–58.

Shinn, M. R., & Marston, D. (1985). Differentiating mildly handicapped, low-achieving and regular education students: A curriculum-based approach. *Remedial and Special Education, 6,* 31–45.

Shinn, M. R., Tindal, G., Spira, D., & Marston, D. (1987). Practice of learning disabilities as social policy. *Learning Disability Quarterly, 10,* 17–28.

Shinn, M. R., Tindal, G., & Stein, S. (1988). Curriculum-based assessment and the identification of mildly handicapped students: A research review. *Professional School Psychology, 3,* 69–85.

Shinn, M. R., Ysseldyke, J. E., Deno, S. L., & Tindal, G. (1986). A comparison of differences between students labeled learning disabled and low achieving on measures of classroom performance. *Journal of Learning Disabilities, 19,* 545–552.

Skiba, R., Magnusson, D., Marston, D., & Erickson, K. (1986). *The assessment of mathematics performance in special education: Achievement tests, proficiency tests, or formative evaluation?* Minneapolis: Special Services, Minneapolis Public Schools.

Smith, D. K. (1984). Practicing school psychologists: Their characteristics, activities, and populations served. *Professional Psychology: Research and Practice, 15,* 798–810.

Thurlow, M. L., & Ysseldyke, J. E. (1982). Instructional planning: Information collected by school psychologists vs. information considered useful by teachers. *Journal of School Psychology, 20,* 3–10.

Tindal, G. (1988). *Curriculum-based measurement.* In J. L. Graden, J. E. Zins, & M. J. Curtis (Eds.), *Alternative educational delivery systems: Enhancing instructional options for all students* (pp. 111–136). Kent, OH: National Association of School Psychologists.

Tindal, G., Shinn, M., Fuchs, L., Fuchs, D., Deno, S., & Germann, G. (1983). *The technical adequacy of a basal reading series mastery test* (Research Report No. 113). Minneapolis: University of Minnesota Institute for Research on Learning Disabilities.

Tindal, G., Fuchs, L., Fuchs, D., Shinn, M., Deno, S., & Germann, G. (1983). *The technical adequacy of a basal reading series mastery test: The Scott–Foresman reading program* (Research Report No. 128). Minneapolis: Institute for Research on Learning Disabilities.

Tindal, G., Fuchs, L., Fuchs, D., Shinn, M. R., Deno, S. L., & Germann, G. (1985). Empirical validation of criterion-referenced tests. *Journal of Educational Research, 78,* 203–209.

Tindal, G., Germann, G., & Deno, S. L. (1983). *Descriptive research on the Pine County norms: A compilation of findings* (Research Report No. 132). Minneapolis: University of Minnesota Institute for Research on Learning Disabilities.

Tindal, G., Marston, D., & Deno, S. L. (1983). *The reliability of direct and repeated measurement* (Research Report No. 109). Minneapolis: University of Minnesota Institute for Research on Learning Disabilities.

Tractman, G. (1981). On such a full sea. *School Psychology Review, 10,* 138–181.

Tucker, J. (1985). Curriculum-based assessment: An introduction. *Exceptional Children, 52,* 199–204.

Videen, J., Deno, S. L., & Marston, D. (1982). *Correct word sequences: A valid indicator of proficiency in written expression* (Research Report No. 84). Minneapolis: University of Minnesota Institute for Research on Learning Disabilities.

Warner, M., Schumaker, J., Alley, G., & Deshler, D. (1980). Learning disabled adolescents in the public schools: Are they different from other low achievers? *Exceptional Education Quarterly, 1,* 217–236.

Wechsler, D. (1974). *Manual for the Wechsler intelligence scale for children–revised.* New York: Psychological Corporation.

White, O. R., & Haring, N. G. (1980). *Exceptional teaching* (2nd ed.). Columbus, OH: Merrill.

Wilson, L. (1985). Large-scale learning disability identification: The reprieve of a concept. *Exceptional Children, 52,* 44–51.

Woodcock, R. M. (1973). *Woodcock Reading Mastery Test.* Circle Pines, MN: American Guidance Corp.

Ysseldyke, J. E., & Marston, D. (1982). A critical analysis of standardized reading tests. *School Psychology Review, 11,* 257–266.

Ysseldyke, J. E., Algozzine, B., & Epps, S. (1983). A logical and empirical analysis of current practices in classifying students as handicapped. *Exceptional Children, 50,* 160–166.

Ysseldyke, J. E., Algozzine, B., Regan, R., & Potter, M. (1980). Technical adequacy of tests used by professionals in simulated decision making. *Psychology in the Schools, 17,* 202–209.

Ysseldyke, J. E., Algozzine, B., Richey, L., & Graden, J. (1982). Declaring students eligible for learning disabilities services: Why bother with the data? *Learning Disability Quarterly, 5,* 37–44.

Ysseldyke, J. E., Algozzine, B., Shinn, M. R., & McGue, M. (1982). Similarities and differences between low achievers and students labeled learning disabled. *Journal of Special Education, 16,* 73–85.

Ysseldyke, J. E., & Thurlow, M. L. (1984). Assessment practices in special education: Adequacy and appropriateness. *Educational Psychologist, 9,* 123–136.

Ysseldyke, J. E., Thurlow, M. L., Graden, J., Wesson, C., Algozzine, B., & Deno, S. L., (1983). Generalizations from five years of research on assessment and decision making: The University of Minnesota Institute. *Exceptional Education Quarterly, 4,* 75–93.

3

Case Study of Ann H: From Referral to Annual Review

Mark R. Shinn

As presented in Chapter 1, curriculum-based measurement procedures (CBM) are used to provide content valid indicators of students' academic achievement. These data are used to assist in making a variety of important educational decisions. As presented in Chapter 2, these data are reliable and are valid with respect to other accepted measures of academic achievement. Importantly, the student performance data collected for one decision (e.g., screening) are related to the data used to make other decisions (e.g., IEP planning, monitoring academic progress). As a result, data collection and decision making are a more continuous process than in traditional assessment and decision-making practice. This chapter presents a case study of Ann H, who was referred for, and ultimately placed in, special education. Both the process of data collection, including the types of CBM measures and the decision-making standards, and the rationale for each of the decisions are presented.

REFERRAL

Ann H, a fourth-grade student, was referred by her regular class-room teacher in November because of academic difficulties. On the referral form, her teacher listed Ann's low academic achievement in reading, spelling, and math as the primary concerns. Concern was expressed also about Ann's rate of work completion in these three areas. An interview with the classroom teacher, conducted by the special education teacher, confirmed the reasons for referral. At the time of the interview, the classroom teacher prioritized Ann's academic problems as in the area of reading, followed by math and spelling. The teacher had no clear explanations for the potential problem(s), though he believed that the failure to complete work assignments was contributing to the lack of progress. He stated that he thought Ann's ability was not a concern and that she demonstrated excellent social skills with her peers and other adults. The special education teacher initiated the special education screening process that included a school records review and assessment in the areas of curricula concern in addition to an interview with the regular education teacher. The goals of these tasks were to (1) determine the magnitude of the difference between Ann's skills and the teacher's expectations and (2) rule out any obvious explanations (e.g., lack of opportunity, poor instruction, hearing or vision problems) for the problem. Should the problem be validated and no obvious explanation exist to explain it, then further assessment for special education eligibility would be warranted.

Records Review

An examination of Ann's school records revealed that Ann had received satisfactory ratings in all academic and social areas from her first-grade teacher. Beginning in second grade, concern was noted regarding Ann's reading skills. In mid-third-grade, Ann began receiving Chapter I services in reading for one-half hour to supplement her regular education reading instruction. An analysis of Ann's biannual group achievement testing results indicated a general pattern of lower percentile rank scores. Whereas her first-grade test results indicated that Ann had earned scores ranging from the 20th to the 34th percentile, her third-grade testing results were consistently in the 14th to 23rd percentile. Reading scores were consistently below her math scores. Yearly hearing and vision screening results were negative, and Ann had a good attendance history.

CBM Screening

Using a process detailed in Chapter 4, Ann was tested by the special education teacher for three consecutive days in reading, spelling, and math materials selected from the curriculum content that typical children in her grade were using. The basic measurement strategies described in Chapter 2 were employed. Each day, Ann read three randomly selected passages from the middle-fourth-grade Harcourt, Brace Jovanovich basal text (Early, Canfield, Karlin, & Schottman, 1979). Her teacher used a tape recorder to record her oral reading fluency and to assist in analyzing the kinds of errors Ann made at a later time. Additionally, Ann wrote words that were dictated to her for 2 minutes from the Curriculum Associates spelling series (Woodruff & Moore, 1985) and completed three probes in math for 2 minutes each. The math probes consisted of one probe of mixed computational probes sampled to represent the Heath curriculum (Rucker, Dilley, & Lowry, 1983) and one probe of basic multiplication facts and one probe of basic division facts. Total testing time per day was less than 20 minutes. The results of the 3 days of testing are presented in Table 3.1.

The results of the screening testing are compared to the median scores of the peers. In a two-step decision-making process, referred students must perform at half the rate of peers or lower to be assessed for special education eligibility. The relationship between Ann's scores and the median of her same-grade peers is represented in Figure 3.1. The points represent Ann's median scores for each of the days she was tested. The solid line represents the median performance of her peers, and the wavy line corresponds to the cutoff scores in each area.

Ann's tests revealed that she performed below her peers' typical scores in all three academic areas. Her percentile rank scores in reading, spelling, and math multiplication, division, and mixed problems were below the first percentile and 28th, 39th, 32nd,

Table 3.1. Results of CBM Screening for Ann H

Academic area		Day 1	Day 2	Day 3	Median	Peer median
Reading	Passage 1	33	16	40		
	Passage 2	41	26	23		
	Passage 3	24	31	25		
	Daily median	33	26	25	25 WC	108 WC
Spelling		67	63	70	67 CLS	83 CLS
Math multiplication		15	22	20	20 CD	24 CD
Math division		6	3	6	6 CD	8 CD
Math grade 4		16	18	13	16 CD	24 CD

Note. WC= words read correctly; CLS= correct letter sequences; CD= correct digits.

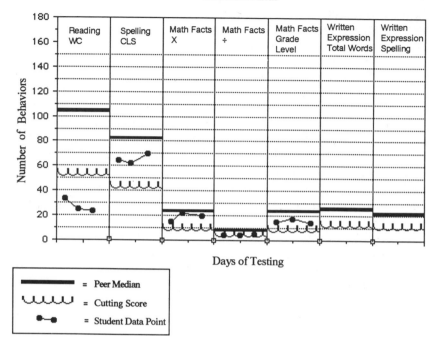

FIGURE 3.1. Results of special education screening for Ann H.

and 26th percentiles, respectively. However, she consistently performed below the cutoff score only in reading. Because the
teacher interview and records search identified no obvious explanations for the severe deficit in reading, the multidisciplinary team
recommended that a more extensive assessment be conducted.

ELIGIBILITY DETERMINATION

Permission to assess Ann for special education eligibility was requested and received from her parents. The goal of the assessment process was to identify (1) possible contributions to the
problem situation by Ann's classroom behavior and/or ineffective
teaching strategies, (2) potential changes in teaching methods that
could maintain her in the regular classroom, and (3) determine if
Ann met the district's special education eligibility criteria.

Systematic Observations

Ann was observed by the school psychologist on four separate occasions, twice in both reading and math, to examine Ann's behavior in instructional settings to identify situational factors that could explain the reading discrepancies. Ann was observed in math to contrast an area in which she performed higher academically (math) to one in which she performed lower academically (reading). These observations were intended to identify potential work behaviors or motivational explanations that could account for the differences in her performance. Reading instruction took place in a small group of six students for approximately 30–40 minutes on a daily basis. Ann was placed in the lowest reading group in the classroom. The results of the observations indicated that Ann spent nearly 90% of the 10-second intervals in which she was observed in on-task behavior. She was oriented to the teacher and appeared to be listening during the teacher-directed reading instruction; she worked independently during the period when she was to complete her workbook. Ann's off-task behavior consisted of brief periods of passive nonattending (i.e., looking out the window or at her classmates). Although she appeared to be attending, she did not answer correctly any of the 10 questions that her teacher asked her across both observations. Similarly, the small amount of work that was completed in the workbook was done with 10% accuracy. Only one of 10 multiple-choice questions was answered correctly. A postobservation interview with the teacher suggested that these sample observations were typical of Ann's behavior. Ann's teacher provided Ann as many opportunities to respond as her peers and used providing the answer as a correction strategy when students did not respond correctly. The teacher also called on students who had given incorrect answers shortly after providing corrective feedback.

Observation of Ann in math resulted in different conclusions. Math instruction was designed to be self-paced in a group of the entire classroom. All students were to complete a series of sequenced worksheets that provided a guided set of instructions at the top of each page. Ann was engaged academically less that 50% of the time across both observations. She completed less than one third of one of the five assigned worksheets the first day and approximately one half of the six tasks assigned to her the second day. The work that she did complete was done with 85% accuracy, however. Most of Ann's off-task behavior consisted of walking around the room and talking to other female students. Three teacher attempts to redirect Ann to complete her work were ineffective in increasing her productivity.

CBM Eligibility Assessment

Using the procedures described in more detail in Chapter 4, Ann's special education teacher tested her in successively lower levels of the reading curriculum. Again, she read at least three randomly selected passages from each level of the curriculum. If her performance within any level was highly variable, additional passages would be administered until a consistent estimate of reading skills within that level was obtained. Her teacher also tape-recorded the results so that Ann's reading errors could be analyzed later. The goals of the CBM testing were fourfold: (1) to determine Ann's normative performance level so that her eligibility for special education could be decided, (2) to determine what reading material might be considered appropriate for instructional purposes, (3) to collect samples of Ann's current performance so that appropriate IEP long-range goals could be written if necessary, and (4) to collect a variety of samples of Ann's reading skills including the types of errors she made so that a tentative teaching plan could be developed. The results of Ann's CBM testing results are presented in Table 3.2.

Ann's performance in her grade-level material was available from screening, so it was not necessary for her to be tested again at that level. Ann's reading scores fell outside the range of the typical (16th to 84th percentile scores) of students of her own grade and third grade. Her normative score (i.e., the point at which she reads grade-level material comparably to other students) corresponded to second grade. She read second-grade material at approximately

Table 3.2. Results of CBM Reading Eligibility Testing for Ann H

Grade-level material	Number of words read correctly	Fall peer median	Fall percentile rank
4	25 WC	108 WC	<1st
3	35 WC	85 WC	9th
2	47 WC	53 WC	45th
1	64 WC	2 WC	99th

Note. Abbreviations as in Table 3.1.

the same rate as second graders in the fall of the school year. To facilitate decision making, Ann's reading scores were graphed on Figure 3.2, which shows Ann's performance compared to the range of students in the regular classroom.

Ann's school district's criterion for eligibility was a normative score of 2 years below grade level or falling below the 16th percentile of students one grade below. Ann's scores would qualify her for special education should the other exclusionary criteria of PL 94-142 be met. Her normative score is represented by the grade level at which her score falls outside the "box" in Figure 3.2. Ann's instructional level was determined to be second-grade material, as that was the highest level at which she read 40–60 words correctly per minute (Fuchs, Fuchs, & Deno, 1982). An analysis of Ann's errors across the different readers evidenced consistent difficulties with both regular and irregular words. She did not employ decoding strategies for words that she read immediately, and her oral reading was characterized by frequent pauses and repetitions of the previous words. Ann did not attend to the prosadic features of the text until she read from the second-grade

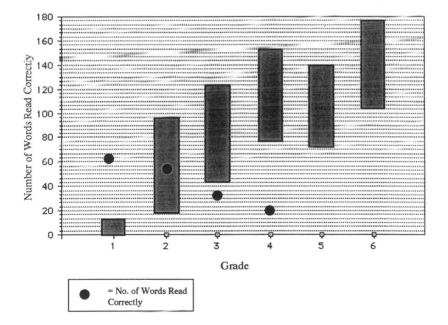

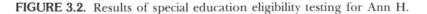

FIGURE 3.2. Results of special education eligibility testing for Ann H.

reader. That is, she frequently ignored punctuation cues for read-ing, such as not pausing at the end of sentences or not raising her voice tone after question marks.

Eligibility Outcome

In determining if Ann was eligible for special education, the multi-disciplinary team considered the wide range of data available. The classroom observations did not evidence any problem behaviors or inappropriate instruction that could contribute to the reading difficulties. Learning aptitude was not a concern, and her reading difficulties were not attributable to cultural or language difficulties or lack of opportunity. Her reading scores and an analysis of her errors suggested a level of reading competence that exceeded the options available in both the regular education classroom and Chapter I. It was decided that Ann would receive special educa-tion services under the administrative label of learning disabilities in the area of reading. Although Ann was performing below the level of her peers in math, the observational data suggested that she was not fully using the time allocated during her math instruc-tion. Additionally, an analysis of her math answers from the screening process and classroom work samples suggested that the work that was completed was accurate. Therefore, the team agreed to modify the classroom math instruction in the regular classroom for Ann. First, a contingency contract was established to set up a motivational program for work completion. Second, Ann's teacher provided 15 minutes of direct instruction for Ann and two other students who were having difficulty with the self-paced instructional program. Third, a twice-weekly achievement-monitoring program was implemented. Short-term weekly objec-tives were specified, and the effectiveness of the alternative in-tervention was evaluated.

IEP PLANNING

Ann's current performance data gathered from the eligibility de-termination process were used to establish the measurement mate-rial and criteria for success that would constitute the IEP long-range goal in reading. The procedures described more fully in Chapter 5 were used. The behavior to be measured was oral reading fluency. The multidisciplinary team used the peer-norm method to write the objective. That is, they chose to use fourth-grade material for monitoring progress. After 1 year of special education, the team expected Ann to be reading fourth-grade material at the rate of her peers at the point of her eligibility (105 words per minute). If she met this goal, her instructional program would be considered successful. Thus, her IEP objective was written: "In 36 weeks, when presented with a randomly selected passage from HBJ grade 4 material, Ann will read aloud at a rate of 105 words correctly." The long-range goal broke down into a short-term, weekly objective of a gain of approximately two correct words per week.

The rationale for this goal was the following. First, both Ann's normative score and her instructional placement corresponded to a level about 2 years below her current grade placement. Because of the team's familiarity with a successful special education program, it was believed that Ann could be instructed at a "catch-up rate." If Ann attained the specified IEP goal, her normative score would correspond to beginning fourth grade. Consistent performance at this fluency criteria also would be equivalent to appropriate instructional material for fourth-grade students. With attainment of both of these conditions, the team believed that in 1 year it would be possible that Ann could be terminated from special education and return to the regular classroom on a full-time basis.

INSTRUCTIONAL PLANNING

Based on the error analysis and the special education teacher's familiarity with the content of reading curricula, it was decided to place Ann in Corrective Reading Decoding B because it provides systematic training in phonics and introduces irregular words. Additionally, the curriculum was selected because it was heavily teacher-directed, a component considered important by the multidisciplinary team. Instruction took place for 45 minutes a day in the special education classroom. For 35 minutes of the period, Ann received instruction in a small group of five other students. Each lesson included a brief teacher presentation, small group choral reading, and individual reading. The teacher used the curriculum and its systematic error correction procedures without modification. For the 10-minute period, Ann completed exercises in a workbook. Unfinished material was to be completed during free time in the regular education classroom. Ann was part of a classroom token economy that was designed to increase motivation and appropriate student behavior.

MONITORING OF INSTRUCTIONAL EFFECTIVENESS

Twice weekly, Ann's reading skills were monitored by the special
education teacher using the procedures specified in Chapter 6.
Ann read from material selected from her IEP objective, and the
number of words read correctly was recorded on a graph. The
results are presented in Figure 3.3.

The solid line represents the rate of progress specified by the
IEP objective. The special education teacher used a goal-oriented
(rather than treatment-oriented) evaluation approach in which
Ann's performance was evaluated using the criterion of change in
slope of learning contrasted to the projected learning rate. The
first phase of the instructional program through the winter break
was successful. Ann's rate of progress (trend line A) exceeded the
team's expectations. After the break, Ann's progress was more

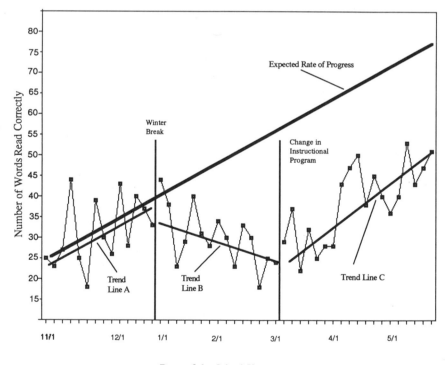

Dates of the School Year

FIGURE 3.3. A graph of Ann's progress towards her IEP objective.

variable, and near the end of the second trimester, it began to decline (see trend line B). At that point, the special education teacher decided to implement a major change in instructional strategies. Based on the observations within the instructional settings, the teacher decided to provide Ann with 10 minutes of supplemental one-to-one reading instruction on a three times weekly basis. This change in programming resulted in a dramatic reversal of Ann's rates of progress as indicated by trend line C, and, therefore, the instructional program was maintained for the remainder of the school year.

TRIMESTER AND ANNUAL REVIEW

Prior to the winter, spring, and summer break periods, Ann was tested on the grade-level materials used in the initial screening to examine her rates of progress relative to the initial discrepancy with her peers. These procedures are described in more detail in Chapter 7. Whereas her initial entry performance was 25 words read correctly (below the first percentile), her first-trimester review score was 35 words read correctly, a gain to the second percentile. At the end of the second trimester, her performance was about the same, 36 words read correctly, which corresponded to the first percentile. Her end-of-the-year testing resulted in 59, a score equivalent to the second percentile. At that time, with some relative improvement to peers and progress towards the IEP objective, it was determined to continue the program at the beginning of the following year.

REFERENCES

Early, M., Canfield, G. R., Karlin, R., & Schottman, T. A. (1979). *HBJ Bookmark reading program: Building bridges.* New York: Harcourt, Brace, & Jovanovich.

Fuchs, L. S., Fuchs, D., & Deno, S. L. (1982). Reliability and validity of curriculum-based informal reading inventories. *Reading Research Quarterly, 18,* 6–26.

Rucker, W. E., Dilley, C. A., & Lowry, D. (1983). *Heath mathematics.* Lexington, MA: D. C. Heath and Co.

Woodruff, G. W., & Moore, G. N. *Working words in spelling.* New York: Curriculum Associates.

4

Identifying and Defining Academic Problems: CBM Screening and Eligibility Procedures

Mark R. Shinn

The certification of students with severe academic problems as mildly handicapped continues to be a major role for school psychologists. This chapter presents a brief review of the rationale for alternative screening and eligibility purposes and describes the advantages of a curriculum-based measurement approach. Research on the efficacy of classification of students as mildly handicapped, Chapter I, or regular education is presented as well. Necessary prerequisites for establishing screening and eligibility procedures—the development of (1) curriculum-based measurement materials and (2) normative comparison groups—are detailed. Finally, specific screening and eligibility procedures employed currently in a number of field sites are reviewed.

THE CURRENT STATE OF ELIGIBILITY DETERMINATION

At the most general level, students suspected of being handicapped are referred to school-based multidisciplinary teams by

Portions of this chapter are based on my 1988 article "Development and use of local norms for curriculum-based measurement" published in *School Psychology Review, 17,* 61–80 (used with permission of the publisher).

regular education classroom teachers. The number of students who are entered into this process is substantial. Each year, it is estimated that upwards of 5% of the school-aged population is referred for consideration as handicapped (Heller, Holtzman, & Messick, 1982). Most if not all of these referred students are then assessed to determine their eligibility for special education services (Algozzine, Christenson, & Ysseldyke, 1982). As a result of the eligibility assessment process, multidisciplinary teams meet, discuss the results, and subsequently decide if students can be certified as handicapped. Available data suggest that students who are referred and assessed frequently (an average of 73%) end up being certified as handicapped (Ysseldyke & Thurlow, 1984). As discussed in Chapter 2 and elsewhere (cf., Gerber & Semmel, 1984; Will, 1986; Ysseldyke & Thurlow, 1984), this referral to an eligibility determination process has been criticized repeatedly and extensively.

CBM AS AN ALTERNATIVE PROCEDURE

Increasingly, the use of assessment materials that are tied to curricula has been put forth as a viable alternative to traditional eligibility determination procedures (National Advocacy Task Force, 1985; School Psychology Inservice Training Network, 1985; Reynolds, 1984; Reynolds & Lakin, 1987; Will, 1986). Most recently, a task force formed by the California Association of School Psychologists recommended the use of a skills-within-subjects model as one of three options to use when assessing minority children. As described by Sandoval (1987), the skills-within-subjects model requires the "curriculum-based assessment of strengths and weaknesses in important academic areas." Unfortunately, to this point, the groups that have recommended curriculum-based assessment (CBA) strategies have not identified specific curriculum-based strategies. As pointed out in Chapter 2, although there are some similarities in CBA methods, there is considerable variability in a number of critical attributes, including (1) standardized administration, (2) reliability, and (3) validity. In particular, if CBA measures are to be used to assist in the determination of eligibility of special education, the measures must be validated for that purpose as required by PL 94-142.

The CBM procedures described in this volume meet these criteria. As presented in Chapter 2, adequate reliability and content and criterion-related validity have been demonstrated. Further, Chapter 2 included the results of a number of investigations

(Deno, Marston, Shinn, & Tindal, 1983; Shinn & Marston, 1985; Shinn, Tindal, Spira, & Marston, 1987; Shinn, Ysseldyke, Deno, & Tindal, 1986) that documented CBM's utility in differentiating students placed into different instructional groupings and handicapped classifications.

In addition to meeting these criteria, CBM procedures for eligibility determination have two other important attributes. Decision making can be both curriculum and normatively referenced (Deno, 1985; 1986) and is tied to the least restrictive environment (i.e., the local regular education classroom). Thus, when screening and/or eligibility decisions are made, the academic performance of any particular student of concern is indexed against local normative performance in the curriculum.

In recent years, considerable attention has been focused on the use of local norms as a decision-making standard for educators (Elliott & Bretzing, 1980; Kamphaus & Lozano, 1984). Local norms are "appealing because they are theoretically more representative of the milieu in which the child is currently functioning. . . . If nothing else a child shares a common geographic region and community with the local reference group that is shared at most by only a small portion of the national norming sample" (Kamphaus & Lozano, 1984). Importantly, it is argued that local norms decrease bias (Oakland & Matuszek, 1977) and, in cases concerning minority students, offer "more information" (Elliott & Bretzing, 1980). With CBM, students are assessed using their own curricula and are compared to students receiving the same instruction coming from similar backgrounds and learning experiences. Depending whether the special education decision to be made is screening or eligibility determination, however, *what* level of the normative sample any particular student is compared to will vary.

CONCEPTIONS OF WHO IS HANDICAPPED

In Chapter 1, Deno presented the philosophical premises that underlie a curriculum-based eligibility system. It is important to recognize that in contrast to prevailing approaches CBM is based on the fundamental assumption that students' "disabilities" are not the problem. Instead, a problem occurs when there exists a discrepancy between what is expected of a student and what actually is occurring. As stated by Germann (1985), "the child's presumed inner disability is deemphasized. . . . In this way, the child's disability is never viewed as the problem/handicap, rather, the problem/handicap is the discrepancy between the child's performance and the expectations for the child." By defining the problem in this way, CBM is based on a situation-centered approach to handicaps rather than on a person-centered approach.

As a result, eligibility determination focuses on assessments that are designed to measure functional educational discrepancies between what a student does on mainstream educational tasks and what significant others wish the student to accomplish (Tindal, Wesson, Deno, Germann, & Mirkin, 1985). A comparison of a traditional view of a typical handicapping condition and CBM approaches is represented in Figure 4.1.

The model on the left operationalizes a handicap as a difference between a student's ability (potential) and the student's actual achievement. This model represents the conceptual notion of learning disabilities and is translated into practice most often by the administration of an intelligence test(s) and an achievement test(s). Numerous technical problems are associated with the intraindividual differences approach (Senf, 1981). These include reliability of difference scores, regression, and problems of high

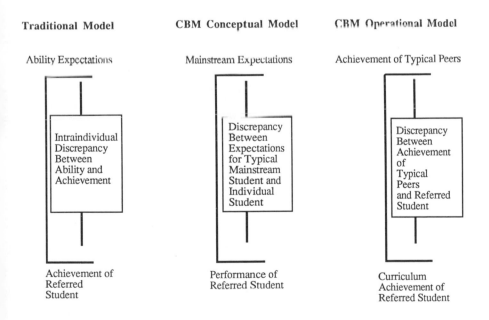

FIGURE 4.1. A comparison of the traditional and CBM conceptual and operational models of eligibility determination.

base rates of significant ability–achievement test discrepancies (Ysseldyke, Algozzine, & Epps, 1983), and, as stated, the problem resides within the child. The middle model corresponds to the conceptual model of CBM. Attempts are made to operationalize the differences between what is expected of the pupil and what actually occurs. This conceptual model is translated into actual practice in the model on the right. The operationalization requires the referred student's current level of proficiency in the curriculum to be compared to the performance of the student's classmates.

As is discussed in greater detail later in the chapter, eligibility determination is based on significantly large discrepancies between the current performance of the referred student and the student's peers. In general, eligibility is conferred when this discrepancy is so severe that the student's academic needs cannot be accommodated within the regular education, mainstream environment, and no viable explanations (i.e., those prescribed by PL 94-142) exist to explain this discrepancy. The actual magnitude of the discrepancy is determined by a discussion of social, political, and economic issues and often is accompanied by examination of the CBM performances of students that schools previously have certified as handicapped.

DEVELOPMENT OF LOCAL NORMS

As mentioned earlier, the development of local norms is integral to the establishment of CBM screening and eligibility procedures as they operationalize the expectations of the mainstream environment. Development of local norms is possible because CBM data collection is both time- and cost-efficient. Depending on the degree of involvement in CBM procedures in special education decision making, local norms can be developed at three increasingly more complex levels: (1) classroom norms, (2) school norms, and (3) school district norms. Special instances such as rural special education cooperatives and educational service districts require some modifications of the basic norming process both in what materials are employed and how normative samples are selected and aggregated.

The development of local norms on CBM is tied to two major pre-data-collection activities. First, a "measurement net," a representative sample of grade-level curriculum materials for each grade to be tested, must be identified and corresponding materials developed. Second, depending on the complexity of the desired normative group, a sampling plan must be established. After these tasks are accomplished, attention must be paid to training the persons who will serve as data collectors, and the data must be collected, scored, and summarized.

Creating a Measurement Net

The establishment of the measurement net, identifying and creating appropriate grade-level stimulus materials for the grade(s) of concern, is a critical task and one that demands familiarity with the content of a district's curricula in the areas of reading, spelling, and math. Scope-and-sequence charts and tables of curricular objectives typically accompany most curricula that are available today and are especially useful.

Two sample measurement nets to represent the typical grade-level materials for first-graders and sixth-graders from a school district are presented in Tables 4.1 and 4.2. The length of administration time for each measure is included in each table. Similar measurement nets must be developed for each other grade to be tested.

In the area of reading, material representative of each grade-level's basic text that constitutes the material in which average

TABLE 4.1. Sample Measurement Net for Grade 1

Academic area	Curriculum materials	Administration time
Reading	Ginn Basal Reader level 4	3 passages, each read for 1 minute
	Harris–Jacobson Word List (cumulative grades 1 to 4)	1 list read for 1 minute
Spelling	Words from grade 1 spelling series	A new word dictated every 7 seconds for 2 minutes
Math	Grade-level math computation (mixed single-digit computational problems)	2 minutes
Readiness skills	Write letters from models	2 minutes
	Write numbers from models	2 minutes
	Say letters	1 minute
	Say numbers 1 to 31	1 minute
	Word reading from pre-primer/Dolch	1 minute

TABLE 4.2. Sample Measurement Net for Grade 6

Academic area	Curriculum materials	Administration time
Reading	Ginn Basal Reader level 12	3 passages, each read for 1 minute
	Harris–Jacobson Word List (cumulative grades 1 to 4)	1 list read for 1 minute
Spelling	Words from grade 6 spelling series	A new word dictated every 7 seconds for 2 minutes
Math	Basic multiplication facts	2 minutes
	Basic division facts	2 minutes
	Grade-level math computation (mixed problems from single-digit to 5-digit, including decimals and fractions)	2 minutes
Written expression	Write a story given a story starter or topic sentence	3 minutes

students will be placed for most of the school year is specified. This information is secured by soliciting information from a variety of classroom teachers, although decisions should be validated by examining publishers' scope and sequence charts and consulting with district reading specialists. As presented in the sample first-grade materials in Table 4.1, Ginn level 4 (Clymer & Bissett, 1980) constitutes the typical grade-level reader for first-graders. At grade levels where there is more than one reader to be read per year, an operational decision must be made. Standards for making this decision include determining what is "most typical" for most students and attempting to avoid floor and ceiling effects. That is, material must be selected that will not be so easy that all students will do very well or that is so difficult that not very many students will do well. In general, however, it is best to err on too-easy material. At the middle grade levels, typical material is more easily determined, as usually there is one text per year. As presented in the sample sixth-grade materials in Table 4.2, Ginn level 12 represents the grade-level material.

Once a specific basal level has been determined for each grade, passages at least 250 words in length are selected randomly using a table of random numbers. In the table of contents, the nth story from the beginning is counted, as identified by the first random number. Additional stories are identified by counting forward the number of stories identified by the second number, and so on. Should the number of stories be exhausted before the required number of passages are selected, the count continues from the beginning of the table.

For purposes of developing local norms, three passages typically are selected for administration for each testing period. Passages written in poetic or dramatic format are excluded. Each passage is examined via microcomputer for readability using a variety of formulas. As readability formulas vary, programs that provide a comparison of multiple methods are used. A microcomputer program that has been used effectively is available from the Minnesota Educational Computer Consortium (1982). Passages that vary considerably (across multiple methods) from the grade to be assessed are discarded and replaced. Passages are retyped to minimize the effects of pictures and type style, and print size is selected to approximate that of the type in the basal readers. A copy with the cumulative number of words on each line is prepared for use by the examiners.

Additionally, a list of words or a passage that is independent of grade level is employed often. All students, regardless of grade level, read this same list and/or passage. Typically, words randomly selected from the Harris–Jacobson Word List (Harris & Jacobson, 1972) grades 1 to 4 have been used. This list is comprised of high-frequency words from the most commonly used basal reading series. A common passage, selected from a third-grade reader when the norms are to be used at the elementary school level, also has been employed on occasion. These independent lists and/or passages provide a cross-validator of sample selection procedures and assist in evaluating developmental trends in the norm sample across the grades and throughout the year (see Chapter 8). The inclusion of these measures makes decision making easier when there is no common curriculum in a district, service area, or at the school level. Student performance may be contrasted to curriculum-specific norms and general curriculum norms. They also serve to evaluate effects of curriculum changes in reading.

To develop CBM spelling measures for use in norming, lists of words are selected randomly from the grade-level spelling series. All words from a grade are entered into a microcomputer, and three lists of 20 to 25 words are generated. Available programs for organizing the pool of words include any microcomputer filing program in which the contents can be programmed for random selection or computer programs developed to create CBM stimulus materials (Fuchs, Hamlett, & Fuchs, 1987; Germann, 1986a). Without computer facilities, random lists from grade-level words can be generated by hand selecting words from the curriculum written on cards.

In the sample measurement net in Table 4.1, words were selected from the first-grade spelling series. In the sample materials in Table 4.2, words were selected from the sixth-grade spelling book. In school districts where there is no common spelling curriculum, words from the same reading level as the reading measures often are employed as a substitute. Words are chosen from the index or vocabulary words from the reader. Again, some districts also assess students of all grades on a common word list to validate sampling plans, evidence developmental trends, and when there are multiple spelling curricula in use.

To develop CBM math measures, a multimeasure strategy has been used most frequently. Each grade is assessed using two separate basic skills math measures and a "mixed" math measure. The former tasks present students with applications of grade-level basic-skill computational problems. As indicated in Table 4.1, first-graders were given sheets of randomly selected problems of basic single-digit (1) addition facts and (2) subtraction facts. The "mixed" computational problems are based on the grade-level math objectives that accompany the district's math series. In first grade, the computational objectives included up to two-digit addition and subtraction facts without regrouping. Thus, probes that sampled from the domains of basic single- and double-digit addition and subtraction problems were created. The probes for the sixth-grade sample are presented in Table 4.2. The two basic-skill probes included basic multiplication and division facts. The mixed probe included problems from the domains of single-, double-, and triple-digit multiplication and division problems as well as computational skills with fractions and decimals. Interspersed were cumulative computational skills from previous grades such as randomly selected problems from the domains of single-, double-, and triple-digit addition and subtraction (with and without regrouping).

The development of these materials is accomplished best by specifying the types of problems to be included on the measurement task from "math worksheet" microcomputer programs that now are available (Fuchs et al., 1987; Germann, 1986b) or by putting together sheets of problems combined from single-skill math worksheets or probes. Care must be given to provide more problems than the best students likely can complete in 2 minutes to preclude a ceiling effect. Basic-skills probes, therefore, include two sides of paper with 10 rows and 10 columns of problems on each side. Mixed computational probes typically include five to 10 problems per column with five rows of problems on each side.

Written expression measures are the least complicated to develop. Generally, a story starter such as "Pretend you are playing on the playground and a spaceship lands . . ." is selected from lists. Story starters that can be answered in a "yes–no" manner (e.g., "Did you like your teacher last year?") or can generate lists (e.g., "Write about what you did when you won $100") are excluded. The same story starters typically are used for each grade at the elementary school level but can be varied.

Determining the performance expectations for first-grade students presents special challenges, especially in the early parts of the school year. Many students have not had sufficient instruction to develop basic skills, and therefore, standard CBM tasks may be insensitive to student performance. Therefore, some school districts have developed CBM readiness skills probes. As detailed in Table 4.1, first-graders complete two measures of tool movements designed to assess a student's fluency in pencil paper skills (Marston & Magnusson, 1988). The tool movement measures require a student to copy letters and copy numbers given a model within a series of small boxes. First-graders also complete the other tasks listed in Table 4.1 including "Letter identification" where students say a repeating pattern of the 26 letters of the alphabet, number naming, where students are expected to say the numbers from 1 to 31 given the number, and reading from words from the curriculum preprimer and the Dolch common word list (Marston & Magnusson, 1988)

ESTABLISHING CLASSROOM-LEVEL NORMS

For most school psychologists, implementation of CBM decision making must take place initially without the benefit of extensive norms. In fact, it could be argued that development of broad-based norms should be preceded by less exhaustive norming efforts to allow for field testing of measurement materials and practice in test administration and scoring. Because data collection is time efficient, classroom normative data can be obtained typically in less than 75 minutes per grade if the school psychologist works without assistance. Classroom norms are based on the testing of a small number of students (five to 10) from a given classroom. The norms that are derived can provide a general estimate of the achievement level of the typical student in that particular classroom. Although level of achievement is important, only gross estimates of the variability of performance within the classroom can be obtained. Therefore, it is suggested that limited classroom norms be used only for initial screening of referred students and for assisting in prioritizing students' needs.

The development of limited classroom norms can be a low-cost, simple, yet potentially valuable alternative to norming projects that require more testing personnel and resources. As stated earlier, the general classroom norm model requires the establishment of a measurement net designed to reflect the curriculum materials of the typical student in that particular classroom. This process is facilitated by conducting a brief interview with the classroom teacher(s). Determining whom to test and how many to test is also necessary.

Types of Sampling Plans

No single "best" method of obtaining a representative classroom performance has been established. At least three methods have been used: (1) obtaining a subsample from the classroom at large, (2) obtaining a subsample from students considered typical of the classroom, usually members of the middle reading group, and (3) a combination of a subset of the classroom at large in the area of reading and the entire classroom in spelling, written expression, math, and readiness skills where appropriate. With respect to obtaining a subsample of the classroom at large, available research (Tindal, Germann, & Deno, 1983) on the adequacy of a sample size suggests that for groups of 40 to 45 students, a sample of five randomly selected students is sufficient, although a sample of 10 is preferable. In their research, Tindal et al. (1983) compared the median scores of sets of subsamples of five, 10, and 15 students from two classrooms of 45 and 43 students, respectively. The adequacy of the subsamples was tested by determining the differences between the highest and lowest medians for each set and by comparing the subsample median to that of the entire class. The results indicated that there was a large decrease in the difference between the highest and lowest median when the subsample enlarged from five to 10 students. No corresponding decrease occurred when the subsample size increased from 10 to 15 students. When the differences between the subsample medians were compared to the entire classroom values, increases in the stability of the subsamples were evidenced when the subsample of 10 students was used versus five students. Again, very few stability increases were noted when the subsample increased from 10 to 15 students. Tindal et al. (1983) concluded that "in general . . . it appeared that in many areas, fewer than 15 students could be sampled with no loss in the accuracy of the reported median."

In Figure 4.2, the performance of two entire sixth-grade classrooms ($n = 45$) in reading from representative sixth-grade material is presented. On the figure, the number of students who earned each reading score is displayed. Each student read three randomly selected passages, and the median value was recorded. The range of scores extends from one student who read 25 words correctly per minute to one student who read 230 words correctly per minute. Most students earned scores between 90 and 150 words correct per minute. The group median was 129 words read correctly, the mean was 134.1, and the standard deviation was 44.2.

To determine how well different numbers of students would represent the performance of the entire group, two different

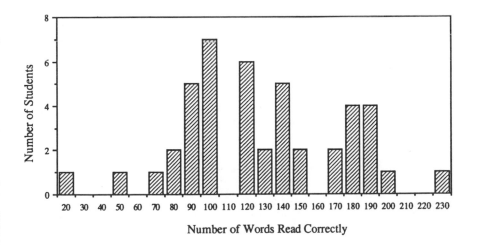

FIGURE 4.2. The range of reading scores of 45 sixth graders.

numbers of student samples were selected (without replacement). The effects of using the median value of samples of seven and nine students were tested. Five samples were drawn for each number of students. The median, mean, and standard deviation are presented in Table 4.3. When nine students were selected (20% of the group), the median ranged from a low of 126 to a high of 143. The median of the five scores, 128, closely approximated the group median for the entire group. When seven students were selected, the median ranged from a low of 106 to a high of 178. The median of the five sets of scores, 123, closely approximated the group median, although the potential for underestimating or overestimating the group median had increased. It appears that 10 students can provide an accurate estimate of the performance of the 45 students. Students can be selected from alphabetized classroom rosters, with every third student participating until the desired number of students is obtained.

The second strategy for developing classroom norms requires sampling from a narrow range of performance. With this method, a smaller number of students are selected, but they are chosen from a group of students who, hypothetically, are more homogeneous in achievement. In most instances, the pupils are selected randomly from the middle reading group or from a list of students that the classroom teacher considers to be typical. By sampling in this way, it is hypothesized, fewer students need to be assessed to get an index of the classroom median. No information about the variability in classroom performance is obtained. Sample norms obtained from the middle reading group from a classroom of fifth-grade students are presented in Table 4.4.

Five students were selected randomly by the school psychologist

TABLE 4.3. A Comparison of Means, Medians, and Standard Deviations when Seven and Nine Students are Selected Randomly from 45 Students

Students in sample	Statistic	Sample 1	Sample 2	Sample 3	Sample 4	Sample 5
9	Mean	132.7	142.0	126.9	138.9	146.1
	Median	129.0	128.0	128.0	143.0	143.0
	SD	38.6	49.5	31.0	40.1	42.1
7	Mean	140.4	131.4	116.9	127.1	152.3
	Median	129.0	123.0	106.0	106.0	178.0
	SD	40.9	42.5	26.2	37.6	45.3

TABLE 4.4. Classroom-Based Norms for Fifth-Grade Students in January

Academic area	Median score
Reading from Ginn 10	127 words read correctly
Spelling words from grade 5 curriculum	13 words spelled correctly
	105 correct letter sequences written
Basic multiplication facts	76 correct digits
Basic division facts	30 correct digits
Mixed grade-5 problems	80 correct digits
Written expression	50 total words written

from a list of 10 students in the middle reading group. Students were tested individually in reading and in a small group for the remaining measures. The five students' median scores were used to provide the estimate of the classroom median performance. For example, the class reading median was estimated to be 127 words read correctly per minute.

The third strategy for developing classroom norms involves the individual testing of a subsample of the classroom for reading and group testing of the entire classroom for math, written expression, spelling, and readiness skills, when appropriate. This strategy takes advantage of the fact that with the group testing, it takes no more time to assess 30 students than 10. The strategy has the further advantage that exact rank orderings of all students are possible in areas other than reading. The variability within the classroom is also evident. The entire-classroom strategy does require substantially more time in scoring, however. Often, this disadvantage can be offset by enlisting the regular education classroom teacher in the project with the intent of gaining more information about all the students in the classroom. Because of the more time-consuming process of individualized reading assessment, estimated at 5 to 7 minutes for a trained assessor using three or four passages, the costs of testing more than a minimal number of students must be weighed against maximizing the detail of the information obtained.

Timing of the Norming

In school districts using CBM, norming takes place on a trimester basis (i.e., three times per year) to reflect the growth in the regular education classrooms. In larger normative exercises, the timing of the norming is standardized. Because of the smaller, less-formalized element of classroom norms, and, as data are not likely to be combined across classrooms or schools, data can be collected on a considerably more flexible basis. Often, classrooms are normed when the school psychologist's time justifies the activities. Therefore, the classroom-norming process may take place only when one or more of the different special education decisions (e.g., screening, annual reviews) must be made.

Collecting and Organizing the Data

Group testing materials must be prepared in advance. They are readily producible via photoduplication or high-quality ditto and are organized best into minitest booklets that are stapled together. The test booklet format avoids the wasting of time in passing out and collecting materials. Most booklets include the three math probes, a prenumbered response sheet for writing spelling words, and an appropriate-sized sheet of writing paper for the written expression task. When readiness skills are assessed, the necessary probes are added to the packet. With adherence to the standardized timing and effective group-control strategies, the group-administered tasks are usually completed in approximately 20 minutes. With subsamples of the classroom, the small groups can be tested in a part of the classroom or in the school library. When the entire classroom is tested, it is easiest to maintain the students in their regular placements. It is recommended that the data be collected by trained school psychologists who are more likely to be aware of the importance of standardized and appropriate test administration practices (see the accompanying section on collecting school district norms).

Because the reading data are collected individually, a variety of methods have been employed. Most frequently, the group testing is followed up with the individualized testing conducted at special reading stations in some other portion of the room or in a quiet hallway. In contrast to the testing in math, spelling, and written expression, where the normative group generates only one sample for each probe, in reading, at least three passages are read from the grade-level material. The summary score of interest is the student's median score on the three passages, as it is the least biased estimator for small samples (Hayes, 1973).

Unless the entire classroom or a substantial proportion of students is tested, there is little need for more descriptive statistics than the median. Again, the median is the best measure of central tendency to use, as it basically ignores extremely low or high scores, and it typically does not involve any calculations. Students' scores on each of the measures are rank-ordered, and the middle score is recorded. If other scores are to be generated (i.e., the mean and standard deviation), assuming the sample is sufficient, microcomputer spreadsheet programs can be used. These programs also make convenient storage media for maintaining and updating classroom norms.

Because of the generally limited nature of classroom norms (i.e., for screening of initial referrals), data usually are organized in tabular form as presented in Table 4.5. The norms are listed on the forms that provide the basis for recording and summarizing the performance of referred students who are screened.

ESTABLISHING SCHOOL- OR SCHOOL-DISTRICT-LEVEL NORMS

When school districts desire to expand the CBM decision-making process beyond the data collected by individual school psychologists at the classroom level, the development of school-level norms or school-district-level norms becomes a logical next step. Understandably, at the most extensive norming level, a commitment of considerably more resources is required to accomplish the task. However, the utility of the data for broadening the use of CBM to other special education decisions can justify the commitment. For example, when there is evidence of considerable school-to-school variability within a school district, it can be argued that school norms constitute the strongest basis for determining the least restrictive environment and, thus, a comparative standard for determining a student's eligibility for special education. Similarly, school norms likely would provide the best criterion for establishing IEP objectives (see Chapter 5 for more detail on this topic). School norms have the added benefit of serving as an evaluative discussion tool for the regular education staff to identify areas of strengths and weaknesses in student performance and/or instruction. In addition to these uses, school district norms have the added advantage of providing a consistent standard across schools for special education decision-making.

TABLE 4.5. Percentile Ranks and Raw Score Words Correct *(RS)* for Fourth-Grade Regular Education Students in Reading from Their Basal Readings during the Winter Norming Period

Percentile	RS	Percentile	RS	Percentile	RS	Percentile	RS	Percentile	RS
99	187	79	130	59	114	39	101	19	80
98	185	78	129	58	113	38	100	18	78
97	174	77	129	57	113	37	100	17	76
96	174	76	129	56	113	36	99	16	75
95	168	75	127	55	112	35	98	15	73
94	165	74	125	54	111	34	98	14	71
93	155	73	125	53	110	33	97	13	70
92	153	72	121	52	110	32	97	12	69
91	149	71	121	51	109	31	96	11	69
90	148	70	120	50	108	30	95	10	68
89	146	69	119	49	108	29	95	9	66
88	144	68	118	48	107	28	94	8	58
87	142	67	118	47	107	27	93	7	53
86	138	66	117	46	106	26	93	6	51
85	136	65	117	45	106	25	92	5	50
84	135	64	115	44	105	24	89	4	48
83	134	63	115	43	105	23	88	3	42
82	134	62	115	42	104	22	84	2	36
81	133	61	115	41	103	21	82	1	29
80	132	60	114	40	102	20	81	<1	28

Types of Sampling Plans

Three basic sampling strategies have been used in developing extensive norms: (1) school-independent norms; (2) school-aggregation into school district norms, where separate norms are developed for both schools and the entire district; and (3) school district-only norms. The normative sampling strategy is based on an interaction of what constitutes the measurement net(s), the characteristics of the local populations, and how autonomous schools are in decision making. School-independent norms are used when there are substantial curricular and/or population differences across schools or when school administrators adhere to strong commitments to models of local autonomy in decision making. Development of school-aggregated or school district-only norms requires that there be either a common curriculum or considerable commonality across schools, that there be some sacrifice in content validity by placing a greater reliance on across-curricula CBM measures (e.g., the Harris–Jacobson word list;

Harris & Jacobson, 1972), or that an elaborate measurement net that samples from the various curricula be implemented.

The sampling procedures for school-independent and school-aggregated norms are identical with respect to the numbers of students required. Typical procedures have involved the random selection of between 15% and 20% of the students for each grade level for each school across classrooms. A minimum of 20 students should be considered. In the instances where school norms will be aggregated into school district norms, a minimum of 100 students total within each grade is highly desirable for determining stable percentile ranks (Salvia & Ysseldyke, 1985). Because the norms are designed to reflect the achievement expectations for regular education students in the classroom, special education students are not included in the sample. Repeating the norming process across years and aggregating the data are recommended when 20% of the school population is fewer than 20 and when the total number of students in the general population in each grade is below 500 (Tindal et al., 1983).

The school-aggregation strategy is exemplified by the sampling plan implemented in the Minneapolis Public Schools during 1983–84 (Marston & Magnusson, 1985, 1988). Twenty students from each grade from each of the 35 elementary schools were selected randomly. A total of 2,720 students was tested on each of three norming occasions. The total normative sample was comprised of 8,160 students. From this pool of students, school-by-school and district norms were determined.

In the school district-only normative sampling plan, it has been suggested that 100 to 150 students per grade require testing. If individual school norms are not to be used in decision making, it is estimated that such a sampling plan can reduce the costs of the school-aggregation strategy by 66% to 75% (Marston & Magnusson, 1988).

Regardless of the sampling strategy, obtaining a random student sample is accomplished most easily via computer. Depending on the type of norms to be developed, students are selected from specific school or school district lists. Some districts have employed school rosters and a table of random numbers when computer technology is unavailable. In these instances, districts have assumed that the beginning letters of students' last names are distributed randomly; every fourth or fifth name was included in the normative sample. Districts often collect information on each subject's demographic characteristics (i.e., gender and ethnicity) to cross-validate their sampling plan; demographics of the norm sample should correspond to those of the population at large if the sampling plan were indeed representative. To address programmatic questions such as how special subgroups compare to the normative sample, districts often include a listing of those students for whom additional non-special-education instructional services such as Chapter I are offered.

Timing of the Norming

In contrast to the classroom norming strategy, more extensive norming procedures require concurrent data collection across grades and schools. Particularly when the data are to be used across schools, timing becomes critical, as a 1-month differential in timing represents more than a 10% increase in instruction. Therefore, the circumstances under which the data are collected are not comparable. Three normative periods are established to represent early, midyear, and end-of-the-year student achievement. Depending on the beginning and end of the school year, testing typically takes place in September–January–May or October– February–May sequences. To the best extent possible, equal time intervals in weeks of school instruction between testing times are maintained. With appropriate methodology, monthly norms have been interpolated (Marston & Magnusson, 1988).

Training and Data Collection

For the school-independent and school-aggregation norming strategies, a number of methods have been employed to collect the data, including using (1) only school personnel released from teaching, (2) paid substitute teachers, (3) paid and unpaid aides, and (4) combinations of the above. The least expensive model has incorporated norming teams of four to five unpaid aides, usually parent volunteers and/or teacher-trainees, led by leadership personnel such as school psychologists. These volunteers are given extensive training and undergo reliability checks, a process integral to all the data collection models. As with any testing procedure, manuals with administration and scoring details are essential. Training in standardized administration and scoring to high standards of reliability is accomplished in one half day. Activities include scoring of examples in each content area, computing interrater agreement, and attending to differences in scoring outcomes between testers. These training activities are followed by supervised practice for all personnel.

Data collection is accomplished in a number of ways, depending on school logistics such as scheduling, room availability, and the size of the team. One person skilled in managing groups of students is all that is necessary for the group testing in math, spelling, and written expression. As mentioned previously, minibooklets of testing materials are prepared in advance so that group testing can be accomplished within 20 minutes. Testing takes place within the classroom or in a separate setting such as a cafeteria.

When data collection teams are used, efficiency is increased when the group testing in one grade is conducted by a skilled assessor who serves as a leadership person, and the team members collect the reading data with individual students from another grade. When the grades are in adjoining rooms or when two grades are tested in one large room such as a cafeteria, the leadership person supervises the reading data collection process while monitoring the group testing simultaneously. Collecting the data individually in reading for large numbers of students is the most time consuming. Some districts have decreased the number of reading samples to decrease the time required for data collection with no significant loss in stability of the norms. With a team of six persons testing two grades simultaneously, both grades are completed in approximately 1 hour. With five teams of four to six persons, one district completed the norming (and scoring) of 15 elementary schools, grades 1 to 5, in less than 4 days.

As reported by Marston and Magnusson (1988), school district-only norms require less exhaustive resources. Unless there are a small number of schools in the district, testing takes place in small groups of students. One testing strategy requires that students selected from all grade levels meet in a separate room. The math and written expression measures are group administered, as they employ the same standardized directions regardless of grade level. Spelling and reading are administered on an individual basis.

In all data collection strategies, scoring is facilitated by having keys with cumulative totals ready for use in math and spelling. It is recommended that reading be scored and recorded concurrent with test administration. Teaming and developing specific skill-scoring specialists (i.e., someone who scores spelling only) can streamline the process.

Summarizing the Data

Any time the data collection process exceeds the informal classroom level, data organization is facilitated by immediate coding for entry into computer. Samples of data organized by grade level can be entered into microcomputer data bases or statistical packages that are becoming increasingly more sophisticated. Scores for each testing period are organized by grade using means and standard deviations. School data are summarized in tables similarly to that presented in the classroom normative section of this chapter (Table 4.4). Additionally, data are organized at the school level by grade in graphic form as displayed in Figure 4.3.

For each academic area, the school median performance is displayed as a dark horizontal line. For example, in School A, the median reading score for third grade is 107 words read correctly; the median number of correct letter sequences in spelling is 68.

When the data are organized into school district norms, data can be presented in tabular and graphic form. One commonly used graphic format is the display of the range of average scores (i.e., from the 16th to the 84th percentile) by grade. An example from the area of reading is presented in Figure 4.4. Two out of every three students in the regular education second-grade classroom read between 35 and 124 words correctly per minute. Two

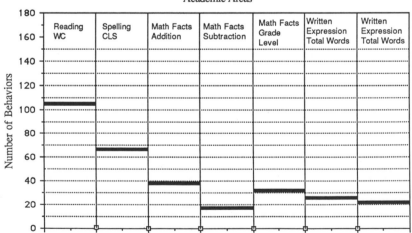

FIGURE 4.3. A graphic representation of third-grade norms in reading, spelling, and written expression for School A.

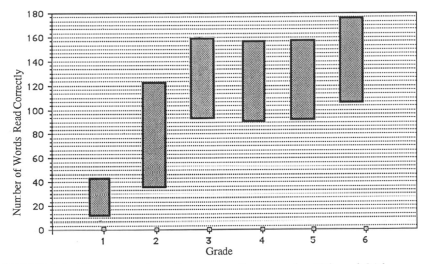

FIGURE 4.4. The range of reading scores (between the 16th and 84th percentiles) in the regular education classroom during the winter norming period for grades 1 to 6.

out of every three students in the regular education sixth-grade classroom read between 108 and 176 words correctly per minute.

When the number of subjects exceeds Salvia and Ysseldyke's (1985) recommended 100 per grade, data can be organized into deciles or percentiles. A sample of school district percentile ranks for fourth-graders in the fall is presented in Table 4.5. Percentile ranks provide normative scores that can be very useful for screening and eligibility decision making.

EXAMPLES OF LOCAL NORMS

The following examples from written expression and reading are derived from two school districts that have developed local norms for use in special education decision making. District A represents a large metropolitan district where Ginn 720 *Rainbow Series* (Clymer & Bissett, 1980) constituted the basic reading curriculum. Data were collected on 2,720 students, grades 1 to 6, from 35 elementary schools per norming period. District B represents a more rural district where Harcourt, Brace, Jovanovich *Bookmark Series* (Early, Canfield, Karlin, & Schottman, 1979) constituted the reading curriculum. Data were collected on approximately 1,000 students, grades 1 to 5, from 15 elementary schools per norming period.

In Table 4.6, the mean performance on the written expression measures are presented for the two districts by time of testing and by grade level.

Despite differences in curricula and student populations, two trends are evident in the total number of words written. First, mean performances across grades increase during the school year. Second, within each district, the total number of words written increases across grades. Third, regardless of grade level, curriculum, and time of norming, the standard deviation remains consistent. Similar outcomes have been obtained for the CBM reading, spelling, and math measures. Data expressed in means and standard deviation can be useful for providing a context for evidencing developmental trends and for examining program effects for regular education students.

Simple methods of representing distributions of scores typically are developed. In Table 4.7, the scores for District A in grade-level reading materials by time of testing is presented in quartile ranges.

TABLE 4.6. Means and Standard Deviations for Grade-Level Local Norms for Total Words Written on a Written Expression Task for Two Districts by Time of Testing

Grade		Fall	Winter	Spring
2	District A	11.7 (7.3)	16.7 (10.0)	24.7 (11.5)
	District B	—	—	—
3	District A	22.9 (10.3)	27.8 (11.9)	33.8 (12.4)
	District B	—	—	—
4	District A	32.7 (12.9)	36.4 (12.4)	41.4 (12.9)
	District B	26.1 (12.1)	36.9 (12.2)	41.6 (12.5)
5	District A	40.3 (14.5)	44.6 (13.7)	46.4 (13.6)
	District B	36.8 (11.7)	38.8 (14.7)	41.5 (12.5)
6	District A	47.4 (13.8)	47.5 (14.3)	53.3 (15.4)
	District B	—	—	—

TABLE 4.7. Quartiles for Local Norms in Reading from Grade-Level Basal Reading Materials (Based on Median of Three Passages) by Time of Testing

Grade		Fall	Winter	Spring
1	First quartile	0	8	35
	Second quartile	2	19	69
	Third quartile	9	52	94
2	First quartile	17	41	60
	Second quartile	40	81	98
	Third quartile	77	119	133
3	First quartile	52	67	86
	Second quartile	79	101	119
	Third quartile	110	132	141
4	First quartile	61	80	87
	Second quartile	87	106	115
	Third quartile	117	135	142
5	First quartile	73	86	98
	Second quartile	102	115	124
	Third quartile	130	144	153
6	First quartile	102	111	117
	Second quartile	130	133	144
	Third quartile	155	166	171

Quartile ranges represent the point below which a specified percentage of the sample earn scores. For example, in grade 3 in the fall, 25% of the sample earns scores below 52 words correct per minute. Half of the sample earn scores below and half earn scores above 79 words correct per minute.

As evidenced, CBM measures are sensitive to the changes in performance of regular students throughout the school year. For example, the median performance of students in the third grade improves from 79 words read correctly per minute in the fall to 101 and 119 words read correctly per minute in winter and spring, respectively. Similarly, students below the first quartile (25th percentile) improve in their reading fluency from 52 to 67 and 86 words read correctly across norming periods.

SINGLE-STEP IDENTIFICATION MODELS: ELIGIBILITY DETERMINATION

In some districts that use CBM procedures, referrals are handled in a traditional way. That is, after the multidisciplinary team examines the nature of the referral and appropriate existing information, due process procedures are implemented. Subsequently, the student is assessed to determine eligibility for special education. This type of CBM model is referred to as a single-step procedure in that no systematic academic screening process is included. Single-step CBM models are similar in that, in conjunction with the exclusionary requirements of PL 94-142, the fundamental achievement testing is made with curriculum-based, grade-level materials, and the student is compared to the norms of same grade-level peers. In single-step models, the importance of quality of the norms is paramount. Therefore, classroom norms based on small samples are inappropriate for this purpose.

The single-step identification model is exemplified by the Pine County Special Education Cooperative (Germann, 1985; Germann & Tindal, 1985; Tindal et al., 1985). As discussed earlier in this chapter, the purpose of assessment for eligibility determination is one of operationalizing the potential difference between the student's performance and the expectations held for that student by significant others. At the referral review meeting, the multidisciplinary team decides from a series of possible outcomes including whether the student should (1) receive a special education assessment, (2) be referred for another school or nonschool service, (3) receive non-special-education consultation, or (4) receive some other type of action. If an assessment for special education eligibility is decided, then the student is assessed using CBM materials. In addition, a direct observation is conducted by the school psychologist "to assure that the academic deficiencies have not been exacerbated by off-task behavior" (Tindal et al., 1985).

Data Collection Procedures and Cutting Scores

In single-step eligibility models, referred students are compared to the normative performance of grade-level peers on grade-level curricular tasks. For example, a third-grader is tested on the third-grade materials specified as part of the measurement net. Assessment is predicated on the importance of repeated samples of the referred student's skills. Multiple CBM probes are administered daily over a 3- to 5-day period, most frequently by special education teachers. This repeated testing allows for a determination of the variability of student performance as well as trend of current learning without special education. Importantly, during the assessment period, the student is tested on a wide range of curriculum materials; these generate an extensive sample of behavior that can be analyzed. As testing progresses, the referred student's daily median scores are recorded and graphed relative to the appropriate normative sample average score. An example of one such graph is presented in Figure 4.5.

In this example, the student earned reading scores of 20, 32, 18, and 25, for the four days of assessment. The student also earned spelling scores of 60, 55, 64, and 60. The solid horizontal line corresponds to the peer median on the same materials. The dotted line corresponds to a cutting score of one-half of the normative performance. In the case of reading, the referred student's scores are consistently below the peer median and the cutting score. In contrast, the student performs close to the peer median in grade-level spelling materials.

Two types of cutting scores have been used in determining a student's eligibility for special education. The first and most frequently used score is based on the discrepancy ratio (Deno & Mirkin, 1977; Howell & Kaplan, 1980). The discrepancy ratio is calculated by dividing the greater academic performance, typically

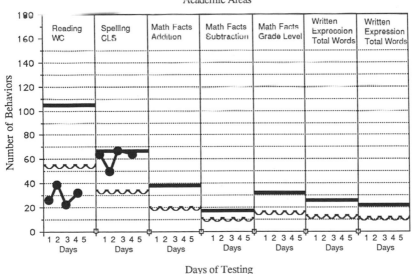

FIGURE 4.5. A comparison of a referred third grader's screening results to school third-grade norms in reading and spelling.

that of regular education students, by the lesser performance, typically special education students (Tindal, Shinn, & Germann, 1987). The resulting ratio yields a number always greater than 1 and has a sign value attached to it. A minus discrepancy ratio is assigned if the regular education performance is greater than that of the referred student. A plus discrepancy ratio is assigned if the score of the referred student is greater. In the example presented in Figure 4-5, the referred student's discrepancy ratio in reading is −2.5, (90/36), whereas in math, the discrepancy ratio is −1.2 (50/ 45). In cases where the discrepancy ratio has been used, the cutting score for assisting in determining a student's eligibility has been −2.0 or greater. A referred student must earn scores of half the peer norm score or below. When used in team decision making in Pine County, this criterion resulted in mildly handicapped placement rates that approximated national averages (Germann & Tindal, 1985).

Research on the specific discrepancy score to use in CBM decision making has been limited. Marston, Tindal, and Deno (1984) studied the academic performance of randomly selected students from regular education classrooms in three states and concluded that different percentages of students conceivably could be identified by using one cutting score for all the elementary grades. Marston et al. compared two discrepancy ratio cutting scores across the areas of reading, spelling, and written expression. For grades 3–6, the median percentage of students who earned scores below the −2.0 cutting score was 7.55%. For the −3.0 cutting score, approximately 3.0% of the population was identified. In contrast, for grades 1 and 2, 30% and 20% of the population earned scores below the −2.0 and −3.0 criteria, respectively. To address these differences, the authors recommended that different discrepancy ratios should be used in earlier grades or that districts accept the possibility that larger numbers of students may be determined eligible at those grade levels.

The second type of cutting score that has been proposed is the percentile rank score. The percentile rank cutting score avoids the major problems that are created by the discrepancy ratio criterion. Percentile scores are easier to understand than the discrepancy ratio, which involves computation and understanding of positive and negative values. Additionally, the percentile cutting score is one that conceptually identifies the same number of students as eligible regardless of the referred student's grade. Therefore, different criteria for different grades are avoided. Perhaps most importantly, the percentile cutting score provides school personnel with easily understandable and debatable criteria about which frank discussions as to who should be served in special education classrooms can take place. In at least one instance, a district's percentile cutting scores were determined by testing a large subsample of students who had been placed in programs for the mildly handicapped on the basis of traditional procedures. Grade-level CBM measures were used, and the special education students' scores were organized by quartiles. Across grades, half the special education students earned scores below the fifth percentile. More than three fourths earned scores below the 10th percentile. As a result, an initial eligibility criterion was established that referred students had to perform below the 10th percentile to be considered as handicapped.

Eligibility Decision Making

After the testing is completed and the appropriate summary scores are determined, priority rankings of the referred student's problems are assigned by all members of the multidisciplinary team. Eligibility is determined by the severity of the academic discrepancies, the priority ratings established by the team, and the ruling out of possible factors that could explain the discrepancies between the referred student's performance and the expectations of significant others. That is, discussion centers around data that are collected that describe attempts to address the problem in the regular education classroom and/or that could explain the achievement deficits. These latter data include (1) health and educational histories, (2) observations of the quality and quantity of academic instruction, (3) the student's motivation and impact of social behavior, and (4) other potential contributions to the problem as identified by PL 94-142.

MULTIPLE-STEP IDENTIFICATION MODELS: SCREENING AND ELIGIBILITY DETERMINATION

Faced with different assessment needs such as large numbers of special education referrals, other districts have conceptualized the eligibility determination process as one of multiple steps. In most cases, the process of assessing a student's eligibility is preceded by assessment designed to determine the appropriateness of the referral by determining if the student is sufficiently different from other students in the regular education classroom that further assessment is warranted. This approach carefully matches the screening decision-making process described by Salvia and Ysseldyke (1985). To be determined eligible for special education, students must proceed through a series of progressively more stringent gates (Loeber, Dishion, & Patterson, 1984). First, students must be referred by the regular classroom teacher or parent. Second, referred students must perform outside the range of the skills of their regular education classroom peers. Third, referred students must perform significantly outside the range of skills that could be addressed realistically in the mainstream environment.

Importance of a Screening Process

As presented earlier, schools refer an average of 5% of the regular education population for special education on a yearly basis. The costs in personnel time and resources to determine each student's eligibility can be enormous, particularly if there is little control over the "quality" of the initial teacher referral. On the other hand, if only a subset of the referrals are tested for eligibility without a systematic process for making that decision, the potential for biased decision making is increased. The role of the teacher in special education referrals has been discussed frequently (Gerber & Semmel, 1984). However, few studies have evaluated the accuracy of teacher referrals systematically. In one district, all special education referrals for students with reading difficulties for 1 year were studied using CBM (Shinn, Tindal, & Spira, 1987). Most students perceived by regular education teachers as handicapped were characterized by extremely low reading achievement. Three quarters of referred students earned reading scores that placed them below the 15th percentile of the normal population. In all grades, the students referred for special education performed at a level of achievement considerably lower than those not referred. In some instances, however, potential teacher biases as a function of a referred student's gender or ethnicity were evidenced. Shinn, Tindal, and Spira (1987) concluded that in addition to concerns of logistics all referrals should be evaluated in a timely and systematic manner to preclude the role that differences in teacher tolerances and biases may play in the referral process.

Screening

In multiple-step eligibility models, referred students are compared first to the normative performance of grade-level peers on grade-level curricular tasks in much the same way as in single-step models. Special education teachers collect repeated samples of the referred student's skills over a shorter-time frame, however; probes are administered daily for 3 days instead of 3 to 5 days within a 5-day period. Again, as testing progresses, the referred student's daily median scores are recorded and graphed relative to the grade-level average score.

The same two types of cutting scores, the *discrepancy ratio* and the *percentile rank* score, have been used to determine whether a student should be assessed for special education eligibility. In the former instance, a cutting score of -2.0 has been used as a criterion for moving the student into the eligibility determination phase. In the latter instance, a 10th-percentile cutting score has been used. In addition to the type and level of cutting score, the type of normative sample used in decision making varies across multiple-step models. Some districts use classroom-based norms, some use school-based norms, and others use the district-wide norms. At the screening level, each normative group has its strengths and weaknesses. Conceptually, classroom norms can provide the best basis for an operationalization of the expectations of the least restrictive environment (LRE).

Because classroom norms can be developed at a relatively low cost in time and resources, they can provide a valuable first step in evaluating a student's needs and the appropriateness of referrals. Referred students who do not deviate much from the performance levels of typical students in the classroom conceivably could (or should) be maintained in that classroom; thus, they would not be suitable for further eligibility assessment. Students who do exceed the skills in the regular education classroom should be engaged in a process that examines their needs and the environment in more depth. This direct estimate of the LRE comes at the expense of differing criteria for further assessment as a function of which classroom a student is referred from. Although some educators would argue that this procedure reflects the important contribution that any particular environment plays in determining a problem, that is, a handicapping condition (see Chapter 1), others who view the handicapping condition as exclusively a function of the student may take issue with the process. Classroom norms have other potential shortcomings. They typically provide only an estimate of skill levels and do not provide an estimate of variability within the class unless larger samples are obtained. Further, decisions based on classroom norms require discrepancy ratios as summary score, since percentile ranks require a much larger sample size.

School-based norms also are tied to an operationalization of the LRE. Because they are aggregated across all the grades in a building, the direct relation to the referred student's classroom peers may be less. Still, with a representative sampling plan, school-based norms can provide very appropriate estimates of both the level and range of performance in the regular education classroom and may be especially important in operationalizing the expectations of the regular education classroom when there is considerable variability among schools within a district. Whereas school-based norms have the advantage of providing estimates of the variability of performance, their shortcomings are much the same as those of classroom-based norms. Typically, they are tied to the use of discrepancy scores, and the cutting score for further assessment may vary as a function of the school.

School district norms provide the least direct estimate of any particular student's LRE, although they provide a strong estimate of the "average" LRE. This general estimate of LRE is counterbalanced by providing the advantage of a consistent standard for decision making across schools and by facilitating the use of percentile rank cutting scores.

After the screening assessment is completed, actual decision making resembles the process used in the single-step eligibility determination model. A referred student's scores are organized in both tabular and graphic form. Based on an examination of school and medical records, and in conjunction with other input from participants, a decision is made whether to assess the student further for special education eligibility. When a student exceeds the cutting score and no obvious explanation suffices to reconcile the level of performance, the student may be further assessed. When students do not exceed the cutting score, referrals may be terminated or sent to another program, or a decision may be made to allocate other services such as in-classroom consultation. The team also may choose to override the data and further assess a student for eligibility.

In examining the effects of their systematic screening process, Marston and Magnusson (1988) reported that approximately 50%

of the students who were referred progressed to the second step of the eligibility process. This proportion was relatively consistent across grades. As a result, there was a considerable savings in assessment time. Further, Marston and Magnusson concluded that the objectivity of the referral review process has increased, as "over the past three years, the student support teams have overridden the criteria in only 10–15% of the referrals." As further verification of the screening process as an effective means for evaluating the appropriateness of referrals, Deno, Marston, and Tindal (1985) demonstrated that the performance of referred students who were not assessed for eligibility (i.e., did not meet the −2.0 criteria) was very similar to the typical performance of students who had been placed in Chapter I programs.

Eligibility Determination

In multiple-step CBM identification models, referred students who are screened and exceed the achievement expectations of grade-level peers in the curricula without obvious explanations are put through a second, more extensive assessment process. As discussed earlier, a handicapping condition is conceptualized as a severe discrepancy between the referred student's achievement and the expectations of others. In a multiple-step model, the severity of the discrepancy is operationalized by determining the magnitude of the difference between the student's current grade placement and the student's normative level in the appropriate grade curricula. This normative level is the point in the regular education curriculum at which a referred student's scores on CBM are similar to those of typical students. The major assessment task is to determine if the referred student exceeds the achievement expectations of lower-grade students in the curriculum to be considered eligible for special education. In all multiple-step models, the criterion for eligibility is based on percentile rank scores and school district norms.

The assessment process requires special education teachers to test referred students in materials sampled from the measurement net that corresponds to progressively lower grade levels. As current grade-level performance data are available from the screening process, a fourth-grade student would be first tested on CBM materials from the third-grade curriculum, the second-grade curriculum, and so on. Multiple student samples are obtained in each set of typical grade-level materials. Correct performance scores are converted to percentile ranks, and both are recorded. The referred student's raw scores and percentile ranks compared to other grade-level peers in reading during the winter norming period are presented in Table 4.8.

As determined from the screening process, the referred fourth-grader's score of 43 words read correctly fell below the first percentile, far outside the range of regular education grade-level peers. In third-grade materials, the student's raw score of 54 words correct was at the fourth percentile. In second- and first-grade material, the student earned percentile rank scores of 37 and 93, respectively. Additionally, the referred student's raw scores are graphed on a figure similar to that of Figure 4.6.

The boxes in the figure represent the range of scores of typical students in the regular education classroom in grade-level curricular materials for the winter norming period. The lower end of the box corresponds to −1 standard deviation (i.e., the 16th percentile). The upper end of the box equals +1 standard deviation or the 84th percentile. The grade level that the referred student's score falls within the range of the regular education peers (i.e., between the 16th percentile or 84th percentile) or, in other words, falls within the box, corresponds to the normative score.

Students in the elementary grades may be determined eligible for special education if their normative score falls 2 years or more below their current placement. In practice, this translates into a criterion of falling below the 16th percentile on CBM materials one grade lower. In school districts that use CBM, specific operational definitions of "significantly behind in the curriculum" are provided to determine eligibility for students in first grade. In the example above, the referred fourth grader's scores fall outside the range of regular education for fourth, third, and second graders. The first score to fall within the range within the regular

TABLE 4.8. A Comparison of Referred Students' Median Reading Scores in Different Grade-Level Materials Compared to Local Norms

Grade-level material	Referred students' raw scores	Referred students' percentile ranks
4	43	<1
3	54	4
2	58	15
1	70	69

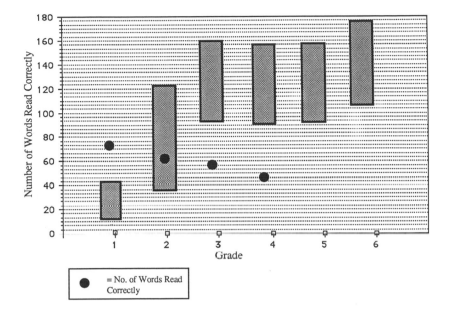

FIGURE 4.6. Results of testing of student through successive levels of the curriculum to determine potential eligibility.

education classroom is at the first-grade level. This level becomes the normative score. The student reads first-grade reading material like a typical regular education student in the first grade.

The specific eligibility criteria may be confusing by the nature of the extensiveness of the testing and how the data are represented. First, it is important to distinguish between the criterion of the percentile score one grade below and the normative level. The eligibility criterion is based on the percentile cutting score. The normative score, which looks alluringly like a grade-equivalent score, is not quantified but is used to signify the general magnitude of the discrepancy. A normative score of first grade for a fourth-grade student suggests that a student has fewer reading skills than a fourth-grade student who earns a normative score of second grade. Both students could be considered eligible for special education, however, as their scores fell below the 16th percentile of the third-grade normative sample.

The second assessment element that contributes to the eligibility decision is an analysis of the errors the student makes in specific grade-level materials. Whereas a major emphasis in testing is placed on determining the number of behaviors the student engages in correctly, the errors on items from the curricula can contribute to determining if the referred student's scores are influenced by a limited number of critical skills that could be taught in the mainstream or are more pervasive and require more extensive instruction. Furthermore, the error samples can contribute potentially to instructional planning. Although there are numerous, extensive criterion-referenced tests available for task analyzing students' instructional needs, teachers often fail to use them because it is difficult to determine which of the many components to administer. Alternatively, some teachers administer the entire battery at considerable time and cost when only a subset of items would suffice. Errors in the curricula obtained in CBM testing can serve as survey-level tests (Howell & Kaplan, 1980) that can be used to identify potential areas that require further assessment with criterion-referenced or informal, teacher-made devices.

Eligibility is determined by the multidisciplinary team using a variety of different kinds of data. Again, discussion centers around the degree to which the student meets the eligibility criteria, the severity of the academic discrepancies as indicated by the normative-level score, the priority ratings established by the team, and the ruling out of possible factors that could explain the discrepancies between the referred student's performance and the expectations of significant others. The team meeting and decision-making process is much like that of the single-step models, although different types of scores are collected, and the information about student performance is more extensive.

Studies of the effects of multiple-step models are limited at this time. In the Minneapolis model, these procedures have resulted in referral-to-placement rates of approximately 25% to 45% (Marston & Magnusson, 1985), well below accepted national rates of 75% to 90% (Algozzine et al., 1982).

SUMMARY

Special education screening and eligibility decisions can be made using CBM measures derived from the regular education curricula and local norms designed to represent the expectations within the regular education classroom. The procedures have a number of advantages. First, important special education decisions are made with respect to what educators ideally know best, their own students and their own curricula. The relevance of norms and testing content is maximized. Second, decisions regarding the allocation of special education services can be made consistently and clearly with respect to how it appears that school social policy currently defines students as handicapped. That is, the same students who are now placed in programs for the handicapped likely will be identified and placed using CBM. However, the process will be less time-consuming and costly and may be less likely to be "subverted" to make students eligible or ineligible, as Shephard (1983) describes current special education eligibility decision making.

This "advantage" does not come without serious potential shortcomings. The most important contributions of CBM screening and eligibility procedures are their ultimate ties to the development and documentation of effective instructional programs. The settings of the effective programs are less important than the fact that attempts are made and documented to improve the academic performances of students with needs. In haste to assess and label children as handicapped, we too often ignore the quality of the program to which the student will be assigned and too infrequently consider if the instruction will be more individualized, different (Haynes & Jenkins, 1986), or beneficial (Shinn, 1986). Clearly, the potential exists to use CBM as a more content valid method of "child-find activity." Instead, it must be remembered that although CBM may contribute to the knowledge base as to whom schools consider handicapped, it is unlikely that anything has been contributed to the understanding of mildly handicapping conditions if, indeed, they do exist. In other words, reliability of decision making may be a necessary, although insufficient, condition for valid decision making.

To address these concerns, it is recommended that CBM screening and eligibility procedures, when implemented, be a part of the "package" of alternative assessment strategies. Such a package has been described in detail by Lentz and Shapiro (1986), where attempts are made to assess the instructional environment in which students are reported to be having problems. Systematic observations and interviews are conducted with the purpose of identifying controlling variables that may be contributing to the problems, including poorly designed or implemented curricula, deficient teaching strategies, or poor contingency management of learning. As a result, it may be more likely to implement successful interventions that maintain more students in the regular education classroom. Further, these same strategies, paired with the systematic monitoring of progress towards IEP objectives discussed in Chapter 6, must be employed to guarantee that special education is indeed special.

School officials will find CBM screening and eligibility models controversial. Considerable discussions will be necessary to determine what special and regular educators consider handicapping in each unique local environment. Cutting scores will be decided initially with great hesitation, and concerns will be voiced about too many or too few students being identified as handicapped. This author argues that such discussions and uncertainty about the nature of mildly handicapping conditions, special education decision-making, regular education's responsibility to the large numbers of students who are not succeeding, etc. can be healthy and are timely. Too often, "handicapped" is defined in complex psychometric or neuropsychological terms that derive numbers without practical meaning. One can question what indeed a 15-point discrepancy between the WISC-R and any published achievement test, corrected for regression, really means with respect to what a student can do in the curricula if appropriate instruction is provided.

Deciding who is handicapped cannot be separated from the practical considerations as to what range of options are available or need to be available to students in the regular classroom with academic needs and what kinds of services special education does provide. CBM can provide "simple," reliable, and understandable procedures for screening and eligibility determination but cannot provide simple answers to these complex questions.

REFERENCES

Algozzine, B., Christenson, S., & Ysseldyke, J. E. (1982). Probabilities associated with the referral to placement process. *Teacher Education and Special Education, 5,* 19–23.

Clymer, T., & Bissett, D. J. (1980). *Reading 720 Rainbow edition: A lizard to start with.* Lexington, MA: Ginn and Co.

Deno, S. L. (1985). Curriculum-based measurement: The emerging alternative. *Exceptional Children, 52,* 219–232.

Deno, S. L. (1986). Formative evaluation of individual programs: A new role for school psychologists. *School Psychology Review, 15,* 358–374.

Deno, S. L., Marston, D., Shinn, M. R., & Tindal, G. (1983). Oral reading fluency: A simple datum for scaling reading disability. *Topics in Learning and Learning Disability, 2,* 53–59.

Deno, S. L., Marston, D., & Tindal, G. (1985). Direct and frequent curriculum-based measurement: An alternative for educational decision making. *Special Services in the Schools, 2,* 5–28.

Deno, S. L., & Mirkin, P. K. (1977). *Data-based program modification: A manual.* Reston, VA: Council for Exceptional Children.

Early, M., Canfield, G. R., Karlin, R., & Schottman, T. A. (1979). *HBJ Bookman reading program.* New York: Harcourt, Brace, & Jovanovich.

Elliott, S. N., & Bretzing, B. H. (1980). Using and updating local norms. *Psychology in the Schools, 17,* 196–201.

Fuchs, L. S., Hamlett, D., & Fuchs, D. (1987). *Improving data-based instruction through computer technology: Description of Year 3 software.* (Available from L. S. Fuchs, Peabody College, Vanderbilt University, Nashville, TN 37203.)

Gerber, M., & Semmel, M. (1984). Teachers as imperfect tests: Reconceptualizing the referral process. *Educational Psychologist, 19,* 137–148.

Germann, G. (1985). *Pine County Special Education Cooperative total special education (TSES): A summary.* Sandstone, MN: Pine County Special Education Cooperative.

Germann, G. (1986a). *Continuous assessment program—reading/spelling.* Cambridge, MN: Performance Monitoring Systems.

Germann, G. (1986b). *Continuous assessment program—math.* Cambridge, MN: Performance Monitoring Systems.

Germann, G., & Tindal, G. (1985). An application of curriculum based assessment: The use of direct and repeated measurement. *Exceptional Children, 52,* 244–265.

Harris, A. P., & Jacobson, M. D. (1972). *Basic elementary reading vocabularies.* New York: Macmillan.

Hayes, W. L. (1973). *Statistics for the social sciences* (2nd ed.). New York: Holt, Rinehart, & Winston.

Haynes, M. C., & Jenkins, J. R. (1986). Reading instruction in special education resource rooms. *American Educational Research Journal, 23,* 161–190.

Heller, K. A., Holtzman, W. H., & Messick, S. (Eds.). (1982). Placing children in special education: A strategy for equity. Washington, DC: National Academy Press.

Howell, K. W., & Kaplan, J. S. (1980). *Diagnosing basic skills: A handbook for deciding what to teach.* Columbus, OH: Charles E. Merrill.

Kamphaus, R. W., & Lozano, R. (1984). Developing local norms for individually administered tests. *School Psychology Review, 13,* 491–498.

Lentz, F. E., & Shapiro, E. S. (1986). Functional assessment of the academic environment. *School Psychology Review, 15,* 346–357.

Loeber, R., Dishion, T. J., & Patterson, G. R. (1984). Multiple gating: A multistage assessment procedure for identifying youths at risk for delinquency. *Journal of Research in Crime and Delinquency, 21,* 7–32.

Marston, D., Deno, S. L., & Tindal, G. (1984). Eligibility for learning disabilities services: A direct and repeated measurement approach. *Exceptional Children, 50,* 554–555.

Marston, D., & Magnusson, D. (1985). Implementing curriculum-based measurement in special and regular education settings. *Exceptional Children, 52,* 266–276.

Marston, D., & Magnusson, D. (1988). Curriculum-based Assessment: District Level Implementation. In J. Graden, J. Zins, & M. Curtis (Eds.), *Alternative educational delivery systems: Enhancing instructional options for all students* (pp. 137–172). Washington, DC: National Association of School Psychologists.

Minnesota Educational Computer Consortium (1982). *Teachers' Utilities: Volume II.* Minneapolis: Author.

National Advocacy Task Force/National Association of School Psychologists. (1985). *Position statement: Advocacy for appropriate educational services for all children.* Cuyahoga Falls, OH: National Association of School Psychologists.

Oakland, T., & Matuszek, P. (1977). Using tests in a non-discriminatory fashion. In T. Oakland (Ed.), *Psychological and educational assessment of minority children* (pp. 52–69). New York: Brunner-Mazel.

Reynolds, M. C. (1984). Classification of students with handicaps. In E. Gordon (Ed.), *Review of research in education,* Volume 11 (pp. 63–92). Washington: American Educational Research Association.

Reynolds, M. C., & Lakin, K. C. (1987). Noncategorical special education for mildly handicapped students: A system for the future. In M. C. Wang, H. J. Walberg, & M. C. Reynolds (Eds.), *The handbook of special education: Research and practice.* Oxford: Pergamon.

Salvia, J., & Ysseldyke, J. E. (1985). *Assessment in special and remedial education* (3rd ed.). Boston: Houghton Mifflin.

Sandoval, J. (1987). Larry who? Coping with the extended ban on IQ tests for black children. *Trainer's Forum: The Newsletter of Trainers of School Psychologists, 7,* 2–3.

School Psychology Inservice Training Network (1985). *School psychology: A blueprint for training and practice.* Minneapolis: National School Psychology Inservice Training Network.

Senf, G. (1981). Issues surrounding the diagnosis of learning disabilities: Child handicap versus failure of the child-school interaction. In T. Kratochwill (Ed.), *Advances in school psychology* (pp. 83–130). Hillsdale, NJ: Lawrence Erlbaum Associates.

Shephard, L. (1983). The role of measurement in educational policy: Lessons from the identification of learning disabilities. *Educational Measurement: Issues and Practice, 1,* 4–8.

Shinn, M. R. (1986). Does anyone care what happens after the refer–test–place sequence: The systematic evaluation of special education program effectiveness. *School Psychology Review, 15,* 49–58.

Shinn, M. R., & Marston, D. (1985). Differentiating mildly handicapped, low-achieving and regular education students: A curriculum-based approach. *Remedial and Special Education, 6,* 31–45.

Shinn, M. R., Tindal, G., & Spira, D. (1987). Special education as an index of teacher tolerance: Are teachers imperfect tests? *Exceptional Children, 54,* 32–40.

Shinn, M. R., Tindal, G., Spira, D., & Marston, D. (1987). Practice of learning disabilities as social policy. *Learning Disability Quarterly, 10,* 17–28.

Shinn, M. R., Ysseldyke, J. E., Deno, S. L., & Tindal, G. (1986). A comparison of differences between students labeled learning disabled and low achieving on measures of classroom performance. *Journal of Learning Disabilities, 19,* 545–552.

Tindal, G., Germann, G., & Deno, S. L. (1983). *Descriptive research on the Pine County norms: A compilation of findings* (Research Report No. 132). Minneapolis: University of Minnesota Institute for Research on Learning Disabilities.

Tindal, G., Shinn, M. R., & Germann, G. (1987). The effect of different metrics on interpretations of change in program evaluation. *Remedial and Special Education, 8,* 19–28.

Tindal, G., Wesson, C., Deno, S. L., Germann, G., & Mirkin, P. K. (1985). The Pine County model for special education delivery: A data-based system. In T. Kratochwill (Ed.), *Advances in school psychology: Volume IV* (pp. 223–250). Hillsdale, NJ: Lawrence Erlbaum Associates.

Will, M. (1986). *Educating students with learning problems—A shared responsibility.* Washington: Office of Special Education and Rehabilitative Services, US Department of Education.

Ysseldyke, J. E., Algozzine, B., & Epps, S. (1983). A logical and empirical analysis of current practices in classifying students as learning disabled. *Exceptional Children, 50,* 160–166.

Ysseldyke, J. E., & Thurlow, M. L. (1984). Assessment practices in special education: Adequacy and appropriateness. *Educational Psychologist, 9,* 123–136.

5

Writing CBM IEP Objectives

Lynn S. Fuchs
Mark R. Shinn

Federal legislation mandates a close connection between goals and measurement. The Education for All Handicapped Children Act (1975) requires that a "free and appropriate education" be provided by all states receiving Federal funds. A critical requirement of this law is the provision of an individual educational program (IEP) that (1) identifies a student's unique needs in terms of goals and objectives (Bateman & Herr, 1981) and (2) identifies "appropriate criteria and evaluation procedures" for determining progress toward these goals (Section 121a.316e).

The close connection between the specification of individualized goals and evaluation of their attainment is highly compatible with the application of curriculum-based measurement (see Chapter 1). Defined within the framework of measurement theory where curricular validity represents the correspondence between tests and programmatic goals (Yalow & Popham, 1983), CBM links the parameters of testing to the goal statements that constitute school curricula. Thus, within special education, where a student's curriculum is specified in the IEP, CBM is used to measure student progress with respect to IEP goals.

When CBM is used in this way, the explicit specification of measurable IEP goals is critical. Specification of a goal precedes and defines the CBM monitoring of student progress and instructional effectiveness. That is, the goal dictates (1) the material on which measurement will occur, (2) the behavior to be measured, and (3) the criteria for judging attainment. For example, if a goal specified that a student would read third-grade material proficiently by the time of the annual review, the CBM monitoring process might be operationalized in the following way. Stimulus materials for assessment of student progress would comprise third-grade passages from the basal text; the behavior observed and scored during measurement would be oral reading fluency (e.g., words read correctly per minute); and the criterion for judging proficiency would be a standard for fluency (e.g., 70 words correct per minute). Because of the close connection between IEP goals and measurement in this process, selection of appropriate goals that are both realistic and ambitious is essential to effective CBM.

The purpose of this chapter is to review IEP goal-writing procedures with CBM. First, typical goal-writing strategies within special education are reviewed. Second, a basic consideration in specifying IEP objectives for CBM monitoring is presented. Third, components of IEP goals are reviewed. Finally, specific strategies for writing objectives with and without local norms are delineated.

TYPICAL GOAL-WRITING PRACTICES IN SPECIAL EDUCATION

It is likely that within the broad parameters of compliance, the letter of PL 94-142 regarding evaluating student progress toward IEP goals has been followed. However, concerns over compliance with the substantive portions of Section 121a.316e remain (Deno, 1986; Deno & Mirkin, 1980). Substantive compliance demands attention to the spirit or intent of the law that documents the delivery of beneficial programs to handicapped students.

Foremost among the many reasons for this lack of substantive compliance is teachers' considerable difficulty with the process of writing adequate IEPs, including the task of specifying goals (McLoughlin & Kelly, 1982; Tymitz, 1981). Typical problems with goals fall into two categories that cover the spectrum of specificity. At one end of the continuum, IEP goals frequently are vague and global, lacking measurable outcomes. An example of a vague goal is "Will improve 1 year in reading." No clear, measurable outcome has been stated, and as a result, both substantive and procedural compliance with the Federal requirement for appropriate criteria and evaluation procedures is not possible.

At the other end of the continuum, IEP documents often incorporate numerous, overly specific goal statements. For example, Safer and Hobbs (1979) reported that nearly one quarter of the IEPs they examined were at least 11 pages long and that goal and objective statements comprised most of these lengthy documents. These goals covered small details that essentially outlined the instructional program the student was to receive. Whereas one might assume that many highly specific goals are preferable to few global goal statements, numerous specific goals and objectives render the task of monitoring progress very cumbersome. With an excess number of goals to track, teachers are faced with the overwhelming task of designing and administering measurement procedures for multiple objectives, a situation that often leads to infrequent compliance with the monitoring requirement (Thurlow & Ysseldyke, 1979; Ysseldyke & Thurlow, 1984). With practitioners' documented difficulty in specifying goal statements that create the framework for the evaluation required by law, a methodology for formulating goals that are neither too vague nor too specific is required. CBM research and field-based practice has attempted to address this problem.

BASIC CONSIDERATION IN SPECIFYING USEFUL CBM IEP GOALS: LONG- VERSUS SHORT-TERM GOAL MONITORING

Given the requisite close connection between IEP goal specification and effective CBM monitoring, as well as the literature indicating that typical IEP goals are less than adequate, a major task in designing CBM systems is to delineate effective goal-writing strategies. A basic consideration in specifying CBM IEP goals is whether to employ long- or short-term goals for monitoring. With a long-term goal approach, an annual goal is specified, and a large pool of related measurement items is created. For example, 500 spelling words representing the second-grade level might be selected as the long-term goal and would be delineated as the relevant set of measurement items. From this measurement pool, subsets of items, or monitoring probes, would be drawn randomly for the purpose of tracking progress toward the goal of proficient performance on this second-grade goal material (Fuchs, Deno, & Mirkin, 1984). The difficulty of the monitoring probe would remain relatively constant over the academic year.

In contrast, with a short-term goal approach, a series of objectives that correspond to steps within a hierarchical curriculum would be specified as the goal. For each objective, a small item pool would be created for measurement (see Deno & Mirkin, 1977; White & Haring, 1980). For example, one could specify an annual goal comprising 12 categories of spelling rules into which second-grade words fall. Then, one would create an item pool to correspond to each category in order to measure student progress toward goal attainment. Thus, in the short-term goal approach, the material in which students are measured would change as they progress through the sequenced curriculum; the measurement material ideally increases in difficulty.

Both types of approaches are tied to ongoing monitoring and are criterion referenced, curriculum based, and consistent with programmatic goals. However, these systems differ conceptually and technically. With the short-term goal approach, the measurement material corresponds better with instruction because the monitoring probes are drawn from the current instructional material. So, for example, if an instructional intervention were introduction of the *r*-controlled spelling rule, the monitoring measure would comprise lists of *r*-controlled spelling words.

Alternatively, with the long-term-goal approach, the monitoring probes are not related as closely to the instructional materials. Although the instructional intervention might be the introduction of the *r*-controlled spelling rule, the monitoring measure would involve spelling words drawn randomly from the pool of 500 second-grade words, only some of which would have *r*-controlled patterns.

Whereas the short-term method relates better to the current instructional focus, a long-term goal approach incorporates a number of advantages. Long-term goal measurement better represents components of the ultimate desired performance, for example, spelling all second-grade words versus specific types of words. The emphasis is on generalized as opposed to specific curricular achievement (Fuchs & Fuchs, 1986). Additionally, the correlation between long-term goal measurement and global achievement tests is higher than that of the short-term goal method (Fuchs, 1982). This relationship was corroborated in a meta-analysis by Fuchs and Fuchs (1986). They coded 18 studies in terms of long-term (at least 15 weeks) and short-term measurement and in terms of type of dependent measure—global achievement test (e.g., Stanford Achievement Test) or probe-like measure (e.g., spelling a list of *r*-controlled words). Results suggested an interaction between these variables. When long-term goal-monitoring procedures were used, estimates of the effects on global achievement tests were larger; when monitoring focused on short-term goals, estimates of the effect on probe-like measures were larger. Additionally, the long-term strategy facilitates data analysis. Teachers can collect and analyze student performance on material representing the same level of difficulty for a lengthy period of time. Data analysis can occur across any contiguous portions of a graph (see Chapter 6). By contrast, analyses cannot be applied across long time intervals within a short-term goal approach because of the constantly changing measurement material. When the objective mastery occurs, the measurement materials also change in difficulty, precluding direct comparisons.

At the practical level, these goal-writing procedures also have different implications for CBM. Short-term goal measurement is easier to understand because it resembles informal monitoring of progress; further, teachers report that they prefer it for communicating progress to other professionals and parents (Fuchs, Wesson, Tindal, Mirkin, & Deno, 1982). However, it also can require additional time commitments from teachers to create new monitoring measures as students progress through the hierarchy of objectives (Fuchs et al., 1982). On the other hand, long-term goal measurement results in time-efficient monitoring. Once the measurement material is identified, little teacher time is spent creating the probes; instead, time is used exclusively for data collection and analysis. Importantly, the data generated can be interpreted more easily (see Chapter 6).

In summary, in recommending one breadth of goals for CBM monitoring, we recommend long-term goal statements. Use of these long-term goal statements tends to focus measurement on the "terminal" or true expected outcome behavior and, relatedly, to produce growth on the type of outcome measure of greater importance to the generalizable functioning of students. Nevertheless, for students with very low skill levels (i.e., students who are at the lowest level of a curriculum), a series of short-term goal statements might represent a more effective CBM structure. A series of short-term goals would allow measurement on discrete behaviors that may be more sensitive to growth. With long-term goal measurement, beginning-level students may perform at a zero level for an extended time.

COMPONENTS OF THE CBM IEP OBJECTIVE

The CBM IEP objectives are written based on a model of behavioral objectives exemplified by Mager (1962). That is, each objective has three components: (1) the conditions under which the objective is to be attained, (2) a behavior to be measured, and (3) a criterion for success.

The conditions component includes the material in which the student's performance is measured, the situation in which the measurement takes place (e.g., "when presented with a randomly selected passage"), and the timelines by which the objective is to be attained. For example, in reading, the conditions might be "In 1 year, when given a randomly selected passage from the Ginn 720 fourth-grade reader (level 10). . . ."

The behaviors to be measured are those explicit, observable, and measureable behaviors specified throughout this book. In reading, a student's oral reading fluency is measured most frequently. In spelling, correct letter sequences written are counted. In math, correct digits written are tracked. In written expression, words written are tallied. Some variations of these behaviors have been employed, however. For example, in reading, some IEP objectives include writing recalls for reading (see Chapter 6), whereas some IEP objectives in spelling also count words spelled correctly.

Finally, the criterion for success is the level of the behavior expected by the goal date (Deno, Mirkin, & Wesson, 1984). Thus, the student who currently reads 50 words correctly might be expected to read 90 words correctly in 1 school year. Often, the criterion for success includes a maximum number of acceptable errors as well. Typical CBM IEP objectives might be similar to those displayed in Table 5.1.

Deno (1986) described the following three-step process of writing CBM IEP objectives:

1. Collecting current performance data: Student performance is measured in the curriculum and contrasted with peer performance on the same measures.
2. Specifying the measurement conditions: A level of the curriculum is specified for measurement, the measurement situation is described, and a date is established for goal attainment to be reviewed formally.
3. Specifying the criterion for success: Based on normative level and/or trend data, or other goal-setting methods, a judgment is made regarding a reasonable level the student might attain by the goal date.

Collecting Current Performance Information

Consistent with the standards specified in PL 94-142, CBM IEP objectives are based on current performance information. When

TABLE 5.1. Basic Format for IEP Objectives in Reading, Math, Written Expression, and Spelling

Academic area	Conditions	Behavior	Criterion
Reading	In *(number of weeks until annual review)*, when given a randomly selected passage from *(level and name of reading series)*	Student will read aloud	At *(number of words per minute correct/ # of errors)*.
Math	In *(number of weeks until annual review)*, when given randomly selected problems from *(level and name of math series)* for 2 minutes,	Student will write	*(Number of correct digits)*
Written expression	In *(number of weeks until annual review)*, when given a story starter or topic sentence and 3 minutes in which to write,	Student will write	A total of *(number of words or letter sequences)*.
Spelling	In *(number of weeks until annual review)*, when dictated randomly selected words from *(level and name of spelling series)* for 2 minutes,	Student will write	*(Number of correct letter sequences)*.

the behavior to be measured has been specified, the conditions and criterion components of the IEP must be determined. Prevailing methods, where published norm-referenced tests provide grade-equivalent scores, are insufficient in that the scores may neither correspond to instructional level nor reflect performance in any specific curriculum (Salvia & Ysseldyke, 1985). In contrast, CBM procedures may use direct measures of current curricular performance that determined the student's special education eligibility. Therefore, the screening/eligibility assessment is linked to goal writing (Tindal & Marston, 1986).

The critical data are the special education student's scores in the various levels of the curriculum. If students have been determined eligible for special education using more traditional measures, then pupils must be tested through the successive levels of the curriculum via the CBM procedures described in Chapter 4. To review briefly, multiple samples of student performance (usually at least three) are collected at each level of the curriculum. Because many curricula, particularly reading series, have multiple levels at the primary grades, additional assessment is done to fill in curricular gaps between the typical grade-level materials. The results of one student's testing in the various levels of the curricula are presented in Table 5.2.

In this instance, the student was tested on reading material from four successive grades. In fourth grade, the student was tested in two levels of the curriculum. In third- and second-grade portions of the curriculum, the student was tested in two separate levels. Finally, in first-grade materials, the student was tested in three levels. In Table 5.2, normative performance in the "typical" grade-level materials for each grade is indicated. In fourth-grade material, the student's score is far below the normative level. As the student is tested in lower levels of the curriculum, where the material is easier, reading performance improves relative to those younger peers: the student's normative score (as described in Chapter 4) corresponds to that of second-grade peers. Depending on the method of writing IEP objectives, different values of the current performance will be used.

TABLE 5.2. Results of CBM Reading through Successive Levels of the Curriculum

Grade-level material	Number of words read correctly	Fall peer median
4B	18 WC	108 WC
4A	29 WC	—
3C	31 WC	—
3B	39 WC	85 WC
3A	—	—
2D	45 WC	—
2C	53 WC	—
2B	65 WC	53 WC
2A	71 WC	—
1C	82 WC	—
1B	79 WC	2 WC
1A	—	—

Note. WC= words read correctly.

Considerations in Specifying the IEP Conditions

After the behavior to be measured has been specified and current performance data are collected, decisions must be made as to what constitute the IEP objective measurement material, the measurement conditions, and the expected duration of the IEP. Most IEP objectives are written to correspond to the time of the annual review. Therefore, the number of weeks that correspond to the length of the school year typically represents the duration of the goal. In special instances (e.g., changes in special education level of placement), the time frame for evaluation may be shorter.

Two interrelated factors must be considered when deciding what constitutes the IEP measurement material: (1) the size of the domain (i.e., the volume of instructional material to be represented) and (2) the ambitiousness of the goal (Deno & Fuchs, 1987). When determining the size of the measurement domain, one must consider the potential variability and slope of student performance. When the measurement domain is large (i.e., one reading book representing an entire grade level), substantial variation in the difficulty of randomly selected measurement materials exists. Therefore, student performance may be highly variable, and decisions about the effectiveness of the program may be difficult to make. In all likelihood, teachers may consider ineffective instructional programs effective when they observe variable performance because, as research demonstrates, teachers describe highly variable performance as positive (Tindal, 1982). Materials from a domain that generate low-variability data are desirable.

Materials from a narrow domain typically generate data with lower variability. However, when using a narrow domain that is consistently very easy or difficult, one must consider performance slope (i.e., floor and ceiling effects). When the measurement material is too difficult, a low or negligible slope of improvement may result. Although student variability will be low, the material may be insensitive to student improvement, and a successful program may appear ineffective as an artifact of measurement problems. Additionally, student motivation may be lower because error rates may be high. On the other hand, when the measurement material is too easy, a rapid slope of improvement may be generated in which student progress is confounded by a practice effect. Furthermore, it is likely that a ceiling will be reached where the student cannot achieve a higher score even though he or she may be improving. A measurement ceiling would require a change in the IEP objective material and, therefore, a change in the IEP objective itself. To maintain practical and logistical advantages within CBM, it is highly desirable that the material remain of acceptable difficulty for the entire measurement period (Tindal & Marston, 1986).

In the case of the fourth grader whose reading scores are presented in Table 5.2, the student's normative performance corresponds to typical second graders. It seems logical that writing an IEP objective in typical fourth-grade material (4B) would be problematic. The domain, at least 2 years in the curriculum ahead of the student's normative level, may be too broad and difficult. Performance could be influenced by a floor effect and could be highly variable. Measurement itself may be aversive and reduce the student's motivation. Most importantly, the material could be insensitive to changes in student performance. In contrast, writing the IEP objective in the normative-level material (2B) could be problematic for other reasons. The material quickly may become too easy. Slope of improvement could be influenced by the student's practice with that material as part of instruction; so if growth were evident, improvement could reflect a short-term practice effect. At some point in the near future, the student may reach a ceiling, and the IEP objective material would need to be changed.

Considerations in Specifying the IEP Criterion

Once the goal behavior and the goal material have been selected, one critical goal-writing task remains. That is, the practitioner must select the criterion level of proficiency. The question is one of how much growth in a particular level is sufficient for a program to be considered effective. For instance, if the IEP objective material is to be level 3B where the example student currently reads 39 words correctly, the relevant question is: Where would the student perform in 1 year (36 weeks) if the program were successful? Because of the lack of available information concerning what constitutes appropriate expectations for special education interventions, it is extremely difficult to select an appropriate criterion level of performance.

Despite the lack of clear guidelines for selecting an appropriate goal performance criterion, research does indicate the salience of specifying a goal criterion that is simultaneously ambitious and realistic. Concerning the importance of realistic goal statements, Brown (1970) has suggested that goals should not be extremely difficult in order to effect learning. This position appears logical, because very difficult goals would be immediately irrelevant and fail to impact the behavior of either the student or teacher. Farnham-Diggory (1972) developed this line of thought. She stated that the intensity with which an individual pursues goals is influenced by the clarity of one's understanding of how they may be achieved. In commenting on the same issue, Prentice (1961) said, ". . . goals seem to be enhanced by the opportunity to see graded series of achievement . . ."; thus, goals within an individual's reach may contribute to goal achievement and related learning. From this discussion, Fuchs and Deno (1982) concluded that goals should be related closely to students' current performance levels.

Nevertheless, a substantial body of research also indicates that more difficult goals relate to greater achievement. Locke, Shaw, Saari, and Latham (1981) summarized the goals literature, conducted primarily with adults in work settings, with the conclusion that one of the most persuasive findings was that difficult goals produce better performance. In fact, it appears that this finding for adults in the workplace generalizes to school-age groups, including handicapped populations. Research on normal children indicates that difficult goals produce better outcomes (Masters, Furman, & Barden, 1977). Investigations with handicapped children suggest a similar pattern. For example, in a *post-hoc* analysis of one large-scale, long-term CBM study, Fuchs, Fuchs, and Deno (1985) found that the ambitiousness of the CBM goal mediated student achievement outcomes: more ambitious goals were associated with better growth. Consequently, research suggests the importance of specifying realistic but ambitious goal performance criteria.

Normative data on either level or trend can assist in setting criteria. Normative reading data, where the typical student performs at a given time of year, are presented in Table 5.2. These data usually are available only for typical grade levels of the curriculum as defined in Chapter 4. As indicated in the table, for level 3B, typical performance in the fall is 85 words read correctly. If the multidisciplinary team decided that performance commensurate with third graders in third-grade material was an acceptable outcome of special education instruction, then 85 words correct would be the IEP criterion for success.

Trend data represent the average growth of students over time.

These data are derived from longitudinal studies and can be used for levels of the curricula where local norms are not available. Marston, Lowry, Deno, and Mirkin (1981) demonstrated that regular education students improve between two and three words per week on CBM reading materials. Marston and Magnusson (1985) demonstrated that students in special education programs for the mildly handicapped improve between one and two words per week on CBM reading materials. To set a criterion for success using trend, the expected growth-per-week figure is multiplied by the number of weeks of instruction and added to the student's current performance. If the trend of improvement of regular education students were selected (2.5 words per week), then in the case where level 3B constituted the IEP objective material, in 1 year (36 weeks) the student would be expected to read about 129 words correct per minute ([2.5 × 36] + 39).

Goal ambitiousness is reflected in the level or trend standard selected. If local normative data are available, then the multidisciplinary team (MDT) can choose from three norming periods (i.e., fall, winter, spring) for any level of the curriculum. The longer the time frame between the current performance data and the normative criterion chosen, the more ambitious the goal. For example, when current performance data are collected in the fall, selecting the local normative score for level 3B for winter would be more ambitious than selecting the criterion score for fall. When normative data are not available, one might use a trend standard for setting a criterion. Ambitiousness for trends is defined by the group on which the growth is normed and the degree to which the rate of growth falls at the upper or lower limit of that particular group. For example, the rate of growth for regular education students is more ambitious than the rate of growth for special education students. Similarly, choosing the upper limit of growth estimates for regular education students (three words per week) is more ambitious than the lower limit (two words per week).

Summary

Under ideal circumstances, an IEP objective would be of domain size that is sufficiently broad that (1) student performance can be assessed accurately for the entire year, (2) measurement avoids floor and ceiling effects, (3) performance generates a slope that corresponds to actual student progress, and (4) the difficulty level is high enough to challenge both students and teachers. The most important factor for selecting a criterion is the ambitiousness of the standard for success.

Limited data are available to suggest clear parameters for "appropriate" and "inappropriate" and ambitious and un-ambitious IEP goals. Nevertheless, with the exception of the ex-tremes of very difficult or easy IEP objectives, the specific di-mensions of measurement (curriculum material and criterion) may not be critical as long as systematic measurement occurs and is evaluated against an objective standard. Further research should provide a more systematic basis for specifying components of the IEP objective.

STRATEGIES FOR WRITING IEP OBJECTIVES WITHOUT LOCAL NORMS

Writing a CBM IEP is possible without local norms. Local norms are desirable for selecting more accurate measurement materials and for writing more precise criteria for success; however, three major methods that do not rely on local norms have been used in school settings: expert judgment, instructional placement stan-dards, and empirical standards.

Expert Judgment

This method relies on two very broad guidelines for writing objec-tives. One, the measurement material must be at least one curricu-lum level beyond the student's current instructional placement. Two, the criterion for success must be higher than the student's current performance on that measurement material. The process is entitled "expert judgment" because MDTs must rely on their judgment in lieu of other more objective data. Although this process is simplistic, the more advanced methods of writing IEP objectives are based implicitly on these guidelines. In the example in Table 5.2, assume that the student was placed instructionally in level 2A. Using the first of the two guidelines, the team selected level 2D as the IEP objective measurement material because it was at least one level beyond the student's instructional level. Using the second guideline, the criterion for success was established at 85 words read correctly per minute, a criterion higher than the stu-dent's current performance of 45 words read corectly per minute. Whereas guidelines' inherent advantage is simplicity, a disadvantage of the expert judgment method is that a specific rationale for the specific IEP is lacking and, on occasion, the goals may be unambitious or too difficult.

One approach to specifying a realistic but ambitious IEP objective is to use a variation of the expert judgment method, the intraindividual empirical approach. With this strategy, teachers initially specify their "best guess" or estimate of what success criterion the student might attain by the year's end. Then, the IEP objective is used dynamically. That is, on a regular basis, a student's actual rate of progress is contrasted to the expected rate specified in the IEP objective. The student's IEP objective criterion is adjusted upward depending on the rate of progress.

The first step in the intraindividual empirical approach after the objective has been written is to represent the objective as a goal line on a graph. This goal line connects the student's current performance (45 correct words) to the goal date and criterion (85 correct words). The goal line corresponds to the expected rate of progress (i.e., the rate of improvement for goal attainment to occur). Then, the teacher monitors student progress using CBM. Using the example above, with the student reading from level 2B, the teacher measures the student's performance in level 2D at least twice each week. After the teacher collects approximately 10 data points, representing about 5 weeks of instructional intervention, a line of best fit is drawn through the student's 10 scores (see White & Haring, 1980). The steepness of this line of progress is compared to the steepness of the goal line. Whenever the steepness of the line of best fit is greater than that of the goal line, the teacher concludes that the student is capable of greater improvement than initially specified in the goal and adjusts the IEP goal criterion upward. Whenever the slope of the line of best fit is less than that of the goal line, the teacher considers the instructional program ineffective and modifies the program.

Fuchs, Fuchs, and Hamlett (in press) contrasted the intraindividual empirical approach, in which teachers raised goals whenever actual performance exceeded initial expectations, with a more conventional, static-goal CBM procedure. In this latter condition, teachers were free, but never required, to raise their IEP objective criterion. In this 15-week experiment, results indicated that teachers using the intraindividual empirical approach (1) raised goals more frequently, (2) employed more ambitious goals by the study's completion, and (3) effected greater student achievement outcomes. Consequently, this intraindividual empirical approach to writing IEP objectives appears to represent a highly viable strategy.

Instructional Placement Standards

Although it reflects the two general guidelines of the "expert judgment" method, this procedure is premised on the identification of a student's instructional placement level and the establishment of how much growth in the curriculum is desired in 1 year. The IEP measurement material corresponds to the curricular level where the student would be expected to be performing in 1 year; the criterion for success is the oral reading instructional placement criterion used to place students in that level of the curriculum. This process matches most closely how current MDTs establish IEP objectives. They operationalize where students are now and where they would like them in 1 year. However, instead of relying on imprecise (i.e., questionable content validity) measures of achievement and grade-equivalent scores, MDTs use the curriculum and instructional placement criterion to write the IEP objective.

The necessary information to write the objective is (1) familiarity with the sequence and timelines of the curriculum and (2) standards for determining instructional placement. Most teachers are familiar with the former; it is desirable that school psychologists acquire this information to facilitate teaming. Currently, instructional placement criteria have been established for CBM measures only in reading. Fuchs and Deno (1982) defined instructional placement criteria as the highest level in which a student reads 40–60 words per minute correctly with four or fewer errors for primary (grades 1–2) and 70–100 words per minute correctly with six or fewer errors for intermediate (grades 3–6) material. In the chapter example, using these instructional placement standards, the student would be placed instructionally in level 2D, the end of the second-grade book, as it is the highest level in which the student reads 40–60 words correctly. For the student to be placed higher in the curriculum (e.g., 3B), the student would have to read a minimum of 70 words correctly according to the Fuchs and Deno criteria.

The next step involves determining how much growth in the curriculum is desired in 1 year. If the MDT decided that 1 year's growth in the curriculum is desirable, then the end of the third-grade curriculum would represent the IEP objective material. In this example, level 3C would be selected. The criterion for success would be the instructional placement standard for third-grade material (70–100 words per minute). The exact value would reflect the ambitiousness of the objective. The lower criterion translates into an average growth of slightly more than one word per week ($[70 - 31]/36 = 1.1$), less than ambitious according to the growth trends of regular education students. The upper end of the criterion translates to an average growth rate of closer to two words per week improvement ($[100 - 31]/36 = 1.9$), more closely approximating the growth of students in the regular education classroom. The MDT selected 100 words correct because of the ambitiousness of the goal and their confidence in the effectiveness of their instructional programs.

The primary advantage of this IEP-writing strategy is its compatibility with current practice. Educators have a history of describing growth in terms of the curriculum. With appropriate, content-valid measures of student performance and standards for instructional placement, this strategy can facilitate teams discussing openly what they think they can accomplish with special education students in a year. The disadvantages are tied to limitations in the knowledge base. To date, instructional placement standards have been confined to reading. Additionally, the standards within that domain vary considerably (Fuchs & Deno, 1982) depending on the reading expert cited. Another concern is that within the traditional educational goal of "a year's growth in a year's time," unambitious goals will be written that do not allow for a catch-up rate. That is, for mildly handicapped students who are 3 years behind in the curriculum, if they make 1 year's growth in 1 year's time, they will remain 3 years behind. This argument is often tempered by the fact that many students historically have failed to make a year's growth in similar time periods, and what is accomplished is a reduction in the potentially widening gap. The MDTs must be challenged to be wary of unambitious goals and to discuss alternative growth rates.

Prescriptive Standards

The prescriptive standards procedure is the most prescriptive, nonnormative strategy for writing IEP objectives. The underlying premise is that the IEP measurement material is selected to generate the best possible data for evaluating student progress. The measurement material is selected based on guidelines that focus on the student's current performance level. Guidelines have been established for reading, written expression, and spelling. Currently, guidelines are lacking for mathematics. Criteria for success are tied to trends of improvement as detailed earlier.

In reading, the MDT selects the highest level at which the following results are obtained as IEP objective material. If the material is at the first- or second-grade level, then the measurement material would be the highest level where the student currently reads 10–30 words correctly per minute; if the material is at the third- through sixth-grade level, the highest material at which the student reads between 30–60 words correctly per minute (Tindal & Marston, (1986) is chosen. In the chapter example, the curriculum material that meets these guidelines is level 3C, although level 4A also is close to these standards. In this instance, the team necessarily would consider the ambitiousness of the goal and the size of the instructional domain. Deno et al. (1984) recommended adopting a criterion of 90–150 words read correctly per minute when this method is used. Alternatively, the criterion for success could be written using the level standards for instructional placement or the trend standards in reading described previously.

In spelling, the MDT selects the highest level in which student currently spells 20–39 correct letter sequences if the material is at the first- or second-grade level or 40–59 correct letter sequences if the material is third- to sixth-grade level. Deno et al. (1984) recommend a criterion of between 60 and 80 and between 80 and 140 correct letter sequences for the primary and intermediate grades, respectively. No instructional placement or trend standards are available for alternative goal setting in spelling.

In the area of written expression, selecting a level of the curriculum for measurement is not appropriate, as CBM assessment is not specific to the curriculum level. All that is necessary is to specify the criterion for success. This process is accomplished by using trend data in lieu of local norms. Deno et al. (1984) make recommendations based on data collected in a longitudinal study of over 500 students nationwide. These data are presented in Table 5.3.

In this table, the average number of words written in response to a story starter is presented for each grade level. The value of the multiplier is equal to the average rate of progress over the 9-month school year. To establish a criterion for the IEP objective for any student, a student's current performance score in written expression is multiplied by the multiplier at the student's grade level. The number is added to the student's appropriate grade-level average score. This sum is divided by two. If the remaining

TABLE 5.3. Rates of Growth for Determining Criterion for Success in Written Expression Derived from Average Growth of 500 Students Nationwide[a]

Grade	Multiplier	Mean of regular education students
1	2.6	14.7
2	1.6	27.8
3	1.2	36.6
4	1.1	40.9
5	1.1	49.1
6	1.1	53.3

[a]From Deno et al. (1982) with permission.

number is greater than the grade-level average, Deno, Mirkin and Wesson maintain that the grade average scores should be used as the criterion standard. In the case of a second grader whose current performance data were five total words written, the IEP objective criterion would be ([5× 1.6) + 27.8]/2 = 17.3) or 17 words written during the 3-minute timing. If local normative data are available, those values can be substituted for the values of Table 5.3.

The advantages of the prescriptive standards method are that they are specifically delineated and may "force" MDT to be more ambitious in their IEP objectives. In one sense, then, it is an easy method to use for writing IEP objectives as the process is objectified. A potential disadvantage is that writing IEP goals in this way can be capricious and arbitrary rather than resulting from well-discussed rationale. There is risk that the numbers take on meanings that are not intended by the authors. The prescriptive standards procedure also needs further research as to the technical adequacy of the standards themselves. At this point, research on their utility in generating slopes that minimize floor and ceiling effects and excessive variability is limited.

USING LOCAL NORMS TO WRITE IEP OBJECTIVES

The IEP process can be facilitated by the use of local norms of performance in the regular education curricula. That is, with local norms, the MDT can achieve a better understanding of the level and trend of their own students in their own curricula. Depending on the severity of any particular student's achievement discrepancy, either peer or cross-grade norms can be used to select the IEP measurement material and a criterion for success.

Using Peer or Same-Grade Norms

Peer or same-grade norms generally are used when an objective is being written for a student who is not greatly discrepant from the typical student in the mainstream classroom. Therefore, the process is used most frequently when students are receiving some type of remedial instruction (i.e., Chapter I) rather than instruction in special education settings. Depending on the norm period used, the student in the worst-case scenario would be expected to earn a normative score 1 year below his/her peers in 1 year. In the best-case scenario, the pupil would perform only somewhat lower than his/her peers in 1 year. This procedure differs from the methods discussed previously in that the IEP measurement material is matched to that of typical peers in the regular education classroom. In the chapter example, regardless of the student's normative or instructional level, if the goal were written using same grade norms, the material would be level 4B.

The criterion for success would be chosen based on the normative median scores from the student's grade-level peers. The specific criterion for success would depend on the normative period selected. In this example, if fall norms were used, the criterion for success would be 108 words read correctly per minute. If the student met his/her goal in 1 year when the student was a fifth grader, the goal criterion would place him/her about 1 year behind in the curricula. The MDT could choose other available norming periods (i.e., winter, spring), however, if they believed the discrepancy between the student and peers could be reduced further.

The advantage of the peer-norms method of writing goals is that it can result in ambitious goals; if such goals are attained, additional outside-the-classroom services may no longer be necessary. Additionally, with the use of norms, specifying a criterion for success is not dependent on the availability of instructional criteria. Rather, actual student performance in the regular classroom can operationalize successful performance.

Using Cross-Grade Norms

In many instances, the peer-norms method may be inappropriate in that goals may be unattainable. In this example, the student would be expected to improve about 2.5 words per minute correct per week in very difficult material. Since the student in our example reads second-grade material like a typical second grader, it may be overly ambitious to write a goal that reflects 2 years' improvement in 1 year's time. When the MDT considers a student to be so far behind the students in the regular education classroom that peer norms are overly ambitious, the team may choose to use lower-grade norms to write the IEP objective. Again, this method is advantageous because the measurement materials and criterion for success can be anchored to the performance of other children in the district rather than tied to instructional criteria that may or may not be applicable to specific curricula.

Procedurally, the first step in writing the objective is to use the current performance information to determine the student's normative score. In the chapter example, the student's score would approximate typical performance at level 2B. Next, as with other goal-writing methods, the team must determine how much growth would be expected in 1 year if the intervention program were effective. That decision facilitates selection of the measurement material. Finally, the criterion for success would be linked to the median normative performance for the measurement material selected. If, for example, the MDT decided that the student would be expected to perform in level 3B in 1 year, the criterion for success would be written as 85 words read correctly, using fall normative period data. Again, a more ambitious goal could be written by choosing the normative scores from the winter or spring norming period. If the student met the goal, the team could conclude that the student made the same gains in the regular education curriculum in 1 year that the typical second-grade student may have made.

The major disadvantage in using other-grade norms to write IEP objectives is the possibility of adopting unambitious goals. When one examines the current performance data of handicapped students, it may be difficult to avoid selection of overly easy measurement material. Clear and open discussion of this possibility may preclude low expectations and allow for more ambitious IEP objectives.

SUMMARY

The importance of appropriate, measurable IEP objectives cannot be understated. This point was stated succinctly by Popham and Baker (1970) almost 20 years ago when they argued that "our concern with the quality of our goals should be proportional to the quality of our instructional efforts." This chapter discussed issues in and strategies for writing IEP goals that facilitate curriculum-based measurement and that permit procedural and substantive compliance with the evaluation component of PL 94-142. The IEP goal-writing procedures typically used in schools were reviewed, and associated problems were discussed. Then alternative CBM goal-writing procedures were presented. First, the basic distinction between long-term and short-term measurement was defined and discussed, with recommendations for long-term goal measurement offered. Second, basic components of and a three-step process for writing goals were reviewed; considerations in satisfying those components and that process were presented. Third, specific strategies for writing IEP objectives with and without local norms were discussed, with corresponding advantages and disadvantages.

REFERENCES

Bateman, B., & Herr, C. (1981) Law and special education. In J. Kauffman & D. Hallahan (Eds.), *Handbook of special education* (pp. 330–360). Englewood Cliffs, NJ: Prentice-Hall.

Brown, J. L. (1970). *The effects of revealing instructional objectives on the learning of political concepts and attitudes in role-playing games.* Unpublished doctoral dissertation, University of California, Berkeley.

Deno, S. L. (1986). Formative evaluation of individual programs: A new role for school psychologists. *School Psychology Review, 15,* 358–374.

Deno, S. L., & Fuchs, L. S. (1987). Developing curriculum-based measurement systems for data-based special education problem solving. *Focus on Exceptional Children, 19,* 1–16.

Deno, S. L., Marston, D., Mirkin, P. K., Lowry, L., Sindelar, P., & Jenkins, J. (1982). *The use of standard tasks to measure achievement in reading, spelling, and written expression: A normative and developmental study* (Research Report No. 87). Minneapolis: University of Minnesota Institute for Research on Learning Disabilities. (ERIC Document Reproduction Service No. ED 227 129)

Deno, S. L., & Mirkin, P. K. (1977). *Data-based program modification: A manual.* Reston, VA: Council for Exceptional Children.

Deno, S. L., & Mirkin, P. K. (1980). Data-based IEP development: An approach to substantive compliance. *Teaching Exceptional Children, 12,* 92–97.

Deno, S. L., Mirkin, P. K., & Wesson, C. (1984). How to write effective data-based IEPs. *Teaching Exceptional Children, 16,* 99–104.

Education for All Handicapped Children Act of 1975. (1975). Public Law 94-142.89 Stat. 773, November 28, 1975.

Farnham-Diggory, S. (1972). *Cognitive processes in education: A psychological preparation for teaching and curriculum development.* New York: Harper & Row.

Fuchs, L. S. (1982). Reading. In P. K. Mirkin, L. S. Fuchs, & S. L. Deno (Eds.), *Considerations in designing a continuous progress evaluation system* (Monograph No. 20). Minneapolis: University of Minnesota Institute for Research on Learning Disabilities. (ERIC Document Reproduction Service No. ED 226 042)

Fuchs, L. S., & Deno, S. L. (1982). *Developing goals and objectives for educational programs.* Washington: American Association of Colleges for Teacher Education.

Fuchs, L. S., Deno, S. L., & Mirkin, P. K. (1984). The effects of frequent curriculum-based measurement and evaluation on pedagogy, student achievement, and student awareness of learning *American Educational Research Journal, 21,* 449–460.

Fuchs, L. S., & Fuchs, D. (1986). Curriculum-based assessment of progress toward long-and short-term goals. *Journal of Special Education, 20,* 69–82.

Fuchs, L. S., Fuchs, D., & Deno, S. L. (1985). The importance of goal ambitiousness and goal mastery to student achievement. *Exceptional Children, 52,* 63–71.

Fuchs, L. S., Fuchs, D., & Hamlett, C. (in press) Effects of alternative goal structures within curriculum-based measurement. *Exceptional Children.*

Fuchs, L. S., Wesson, C., Tindal, G., Mirkin, P. K., & Deno, S. L. (1982). *Instructional changes, student performance, and teacher preferences: The effects of specific measurement and evaluation procedures* (Research Report No. 64). Minneapolis: University of Minnesota Institute for Research on Learning Disabilities.

Locke, E. A., Shaw, K. N., Saari, L. M., & Latham, G. P. (1981). Goal setting and task performance: 1969–1980. *Psychological Bulletin, 90,* 125–152.

Mager, R. F. (1962). *Preparing instructional objectives.* Palo Alto, CA: Fearon Publishers.

Marston, D., & Magnusson, D. (1985). Implementing curriculum-based measurement in special and regular education settings. *Exceptional Children, 52,* 266–276.

Marston, D., Lowry, L., Deno, S. L., & Mirkin, P. K. (1981). *An analysis of learning trends in simple measures of reading, spelling, and written expression: A longitudinal study* (Research Report No. 49). Minneapolis: University of Minnesota Institute for Research on Learning Disabilities.

Masters, J. C., Furman, W., & Barden, R. C. (1977). Effects of achievement standards, tangible rewards, and self-dispensed evaluations on children's task mastery. *Child Development, 48,* 217–224.

McLoughlin, J., & Kelly, D. (1982). Issues facing the resource teacher. *Learning Disability Quarterly, 5,* 58–64.

Popham, W. J., & Baker, E. L. (1970). *Systematic instruction.* Englewood Cliffs, NJ: Prentice-Hall.

Prentice, W. C. (1961). Some cognitive aspects of motivation. *American Psychologist, 16,* 503–511.

Safer, N., & Hobbs, V. (1979). Developing, implementing, and evaluating individualized educational programs. *JWK International.*

Salvia, J., & Ysseldyke, J. E. (1985). *Assessment in special and remedial education* (3rd ed.). Boston: Houghton Mifflin.

Thurlow, M. L., & Ysseldyke, J. E. (1979). Current assessment and decision-making practices in model LD programs. *Learning Disability Quarterly, 2,* 15–24.

Tindal, G. (1982). Factors influencing the use of time series data for evaluating instructional programs. Unpublished doctoral dissertation, Minneapolis: University of Minnesota.

Tindal, G., & Marston, D. (1986). Approaches to assessment. In J. Torgeson & B. Wong (Eds.) *Psychological and educational perspectives in learning disabilities* (pp. 55–84). Boston: Academic Press.

Tymitz, B. (1981). Teacher performance on IEP instructional planning tasks. *Exceptional Children, 48,* 258–260.

White, O. R., & Haring, N. G. (1980). *Exceptional teaching* (2nd ed.). Columbus, OH: Merrill.

Yalow, E., & Popham, W. J. (1983). Content validity at the crossroads. *Educational Researcher, 18,* 10–14, 21.

Ysseldyke, J. E., & Thurlow, M. L. (1984). Assessment practices in special education: Adequacy and appropriateness. *Educational Psychologist, 9,* 123–136.

6

Evaluating Solutions Monitoring Progress and Revising Intervention Plans

Lynn S. Fuchs

Curriculum-based measurement (CBM) can be employed to monitor the progress of special and general education students and to evaluate and formatively develop instructional programs. With CBM progress assessment and program development, teachers routinely measure student progress on curricular material representing goal-level difficulty (i.e., the level of material at which the teacher wants the student to be proficient by year's end). When measurement indicates that student progress toward proficiency on that material is inadequate, practitioners modify instructional programs in an attempt to improve academic gains.

The purpose of this chapter is to discuss CBM as it is conceptualized and employed within the monitoring and program development phase of assessment. The legal, logical, and empirical rationales for CBM monitoring are discussed. Then, issues in designing effective CBM monitoring programs are outlined, and a prototypical CBM monitoring system is presented with a brief review of the corresponding research base supporting the prototype. Next, a case study illustrates the use of the CBM monitoring prototype. Finally, future directions for CBM monitoring are discussed.

Portions of research described in this chapter were supported by Grant No. G008530198 from the U.S. Department of Education, Office of Special Education. Statements should not be interpreted as offical agency positions.

RATIONALE FOR CBM MONITORING

Legal Imperatives

At least three arguments support the use of CBM monitoring systems. The first is legal. The individual education program (IEP) mandate of PL 94-142 requires special educators to specify long-term goals, short-term objectives, and "appropriate criteria and evaluation procedures" (Section 121a.316e) for monitoring students' attainment of objectives. Since the intent of this legislation was to encourage development of systematic data bases to document student progress toward goal attainment, the IEP mandate requires an ongoing and curriculum-based (i.e., goal-oriented) approach to progress evaluation. Thus, Federal law supports CBM monitoring systems for progress monitoring and program development.

Logical

A second rationale for CBM monitoring is logical. As presented in Chapter 1, a basic assumption in special education is that individualized instruction improves student achievement (see L. Fuchs & Fuchs, 1986). The prevailing and pervasive approach to developing these individualized instructional programs relies on aptitude–treatment interaction (ATI) conceptualization and methodology. Proponents of ATI presume that learner characteristics, or aptitudes, interact predictably with different instructional programs, or treatments, to produce comparatively strong student learning. Thus, with ATI, the development of instructional programs is weighted heavily on preinstructional assessment; instructional development is derived from prior explications of learner characteristics. This is a deductive approach to formulating educational programs.

This perspective has fostered research on learner characteristics (see Snow & Lohman, 1984), models of instruction (see Lloyd, 1984), and their interactions. Moreover, the basic and predominant diagnostic–prescriptive model of instructional planning practice within the field is borrowed from an ATI framework. Diagnosticians administer batteries of aptitude and achievement measures to specify instructional programs that match pupils' learning styles, cognitive abilities, and achievement levels. Regardless of whether these assessments incorporate (1) comprehensive ability measurements to identify what instructional strategies to employ or (2) extensive task analyses and achievement measures to identify which skills to address (see Deno, 1986), the paradigm remains the same: deductive, static, and predictive. The implicit assumption of the ATI approach is that the identification of which skills are relevant and which instructional strategies are appropriate precludes the need for ongoing evaluation of student progress. If one correctly matches the learner style with the right treatment, one assumes that treatment success is guaranteed.

Despite the prevalence of the ATI approach within special education practice, several important problems in basing educational programs on initial diagnoses of learner characteristics have been identified. First, incomplete conceptualizations of students' cognitive abilities exist (Ysseldyke, 1979), and available tests of corresponding abilities tend to be psychometrically problematic (Salvia & Ysseldyke, 1985). Second, evidence indicates that the manner in which these tests often are administered (i.e., in one sitting by an unfamiliar examiner) may discriminate systematically against handicapped students (D. Fuchs & Fuchs, 1986; D. Fuchs, Fuchs, Power, & Dailey, 1985). Third, knowledge about how learner and teacher characteristics interact with educational treatments and classroom environments is incomplete (Ysseldyke, 1979). These problems probably contribute to research findings documenting the failure of ATI approaches in specifying effective instructional programs (see Lloyd, 1984).

Although the lack of success associated with the ATI approach, especially in special education, has led some to reject all individually tailored instructional programs (see Lloyd, 1984), an alternative approach for evaluating the effectiveness of interventions is borrowed from single-subject, time-series methodology, and CBM monitoring is rooted in this alternative approach. Whereas ATI methods emphasize the importance of describing salient learner characteristics and/or abilities, CBM monitoring focuses on ongoing, direct evaluation and modification of implemented programs. The CBM monitoring involves routine, systematic data collection on measures derived from curricular goals. This measurement generates a data base with which the effectiveness of instructional hypotheses concerning effective practice for a given individual can be tested empirically and revised as necessary. Thus, CBM monitoring is an inductive and dynamic, rather than deductive and static, approach to developing instructional programs.

For the following reasons, then, CBM monitoring is a logically appealing alternative to deductive methods of program development. First, its inductive nature avoids reliance on initial diagnoses of learner characteristics when conceptualizations of the relationships between abilities and treatments are incomplete. Second, CBM procedures demonstrate technically strong characteristics (see Chapters 1 and 2); one would hope that more adequate data bases result in improved pedagogical decisions. Finally and most important, CBM treats initial programs as instructional hypotheses, which are modified in response to actual pupil progress. This process appears to increase the probability that programs developed with CBM monitoring will improve student achievement.

Empirical Rationale for Monitoring

These logical analyses of the advantages of CBM tend to be supported by research. Ongoing, systematic pupil progress monitoring, in general, is associated strongly with effective general (e.g., Eubanks & Levine, 1983; Hoffman & Rutherford, 1984) and special education practice (Gersten, Carnine, & White, 1984; Goodman, 1985; Peterson, Albert, Foxworth, Cox, & Tilley, 1985; Rieth, Polsgrove, & Semmel, 1981). A recent meta-analysis (L. Fuchs & Fuchs, 1986a) estimated the effect magnitude of ongoing monitoring to be 0.70. This finding indicates that, as presented within the context of the standard normal curve and an achievement test scale with a population mean of 100 and standard deviation of 15, the use of ongoing monitoring systems can be expected to raise the typical achievement score from 100.0 to 110.5, or from the 50th to the 76th percentile.

Additionally, CBM monitoring procedures have been associated with improved educational outcomes. For example, with respect to teacher decision making, L. Fuchs, Deno, and Mirkin (1984) found that a group of New York City teachers who used CBM monitoring in reading were more realistic about, knowledgeable concerning, and responsive to student progress. More recent work (L. Fuchs, Fuchs, & Stecker, in press) indicates that teachers who employ CBM to monitor their students' reading growth (1) use more specific, acceptable achievement goals, (2) are more realistic and less optimistic about goal attainment, (3) cite more objective and frequent data sources for determining the adequacy of student progress and for deciding whether program modifications are necessary, and (4) modify student programs more frequently. Additionally, direct classroom observations (L. Fuchs, Deno, & Mirkin, 1984) suggest that instructional programs provided by teachers using CBM monitoring may be superior to programs developed by teachers employing conventional special education practice in terms of effective instructional variables.

In terms of student achievement, L. Fuchs, Deno, & Mirkin, (1984) demonstrated that CBM monitoring produces better student outcomes, not only when indexed by probe-like measures but also as evidenced on more global achievement tests of decoding and reading comprehension. More recently, L. Fuchs and D. Fuchs (1987a) found that teachers who employed CBM monitoring in math, spelling, and reading could effect greater academic growth than control teachers. Additionally and perhaps relatedly, students whose performance was monitored systematically with CBM appeared to know more about their own goals and their progress toward those goals (L. Fuchs, Deno, & Mirkin, 1984; L. Fuchs, Fuchs, & Butterworth, in press). Consequently, a data base supports the use of CBM monitoring to assist teachers in realizing positive educational outcomes with mildly to moderately handicapped students in their classrooms.

ISSUES IN DESIGNING EFFECTIVE CBM MONITORING SYSTEMS

Although research indicates that CBM monitoring can improve educational outcomes with handicapped individuals, a long-term research program also suggests that specific dimensions (e.g., graphing conventions, measurement duration, methods of data analysis) of monitoring systems can mediate those effects. Therefore, effective CBM monitoring is linked with a number of salient features. A decision matrix (see Deno & Fuchs, 1987) has been utilized within this research program to guide the specification of these essential components. Additionally, this decision matrix can be employed by practitioners to specify effective CBM monitoring systems.

As shown in Table 6.1, this decision matrix for specifying dimensions of a CBM monitoring program comprises three rows and three columns. The rows of the matrix list broad, critical areas for designing a CBM monitoring program. These topics are (1) what behavior to measure, (2) how to conduct the measurement, and (3) how to use data once they are collected. The "what to measure" question addresses the issue of which behaviors with what material represent critical indicators of pupil performance and, therefore, should be monitored over time. The "how to measure" question concerns the methodology of measurement, including test duration, frequency, administration, and scoring. The "how to use data" question involves issues of data display and data-evaluation procedures.

The columns of the matrix specify considerations in selecting among alternative CBM monitoring procedures. First, technical questions must be considered, including (1) the reliability or consistency of the pupil performance scores and of the decision-making procedures, (2) the extent to which the measurement and evaluation system reflects the true construct, and (3) the sensitivity or responsiveness of the system to changes in achievement. A second set of considerations concerns the effectiveness of CBM system dimensions, or how well the procedures actually result in increases in student growth and improvements in teacher decision making. The third consideration addresses the feasibility or logistics for teachers in implementing CBM monitoring.

The intersection of the three critical questions in designing CBM monitoring systems and the three considerations in discriminating among alternatives results in nine matrix cells. In these cells, the technical, effectiveness, and logistic features, respectively, for alternative measurement behaviors, measurement methodologies, and data display and evaluation procedures are considered in turn. The questions within the matrix cells are listed in Table 6.2.

TABLE 6.1. Decision-Making Matrix[a]

	Considerations		
Questions	Technical	Instructional	Efficiency
What to measure	T-1	I-1	E-1
How to measure	T-2	I-2	E-2
How to use data	T-3	I-3	E-3

[a]Codes within cells correspond to questions listed in Table 6.2.

PROTOTYPICAL CBM MONITORING SYSTEM IN READING

To exemplify the use of the matrix in developing a CBM monitoring program, a prototypical monitoring system in the area of reading is presented. Reading was selected as the focus of this section because research indicates that reading is the most common problem area in the schools today. The reading-monitoring system is described, and a brief presentation of supporting research is included. The three broad column questions serve as the organizational scheme for presenting this CBM monitoring prototype. The reader is directed to the Appendix for information concerning monitoring systems in spelling, math, and written expression.

TABLE 6.2. Broad Questions within Decision-Making Matrix Cells

---

Technical
- T-1: *What to measure:* What behaviors clearly index growth and are responsive to the effects of instruction?
- T-2: *How to measure:* What measurement procedures generate reliable and valid data that are sensitive to short- and long-term growth?
- T-3: *How to use data:* How should data be summarized, displayed, analyzed, and interpreted to insure reliable and valid decision making?

Instructional
- I-1: *What to measure:* Measurement of what behaviors relates to improved teacher decision making and student achievement?
- I-2: *How to measure:* What measurement procedures result in improved teacher decision making and student achievement?
- I-3: *How to use data:* What data summarization, display, analysis, and interpretation methods are associated with improved teacher decision making and student achievement?

Efficiency
- E-1: *What to measure:* What measurement behaviors are easiest and least time consuming for teachers to employ?
- E-2: *How to measure:* What measurement procedures are most efficient and least intrusive?
- E-3: *How to use data:* What data summarization, display, analysis, and interpretation methods are most efficient and cost-effective?

WHAT TO MEASURE

What Behavior

In designing CBM monitoring systems, one first must consider the focus of measurement, or "what to measure." Because CBM monitoring is implemented on a more frequent basis than traditional assessment, it requires a significant time commitment from practitioners. Consequently, the behavior to be measured must meet certain practical criteria. Among important practical considerations mentioned by Deno, Mirkin, and Chiang (1982) are ease in administration, availability of multiple alternate forms, and cost and time efficiency. Beyond practical features, the behavior must reflect student growth in reading accurately, and teachers' monitoring of this behavior should produce greater academic achievement on criterion measures than conventional special education without systematic monitoring.

Measures derived from curricular materials are inexpensive to produce, and multiple alternate forms are available. They can be administered in short periods of time. Moreover, the curricular validity of such informal measurement is strong. In the area of reading comprehension, potentially useful CBM measurement strategies include question-answering tests, recall procedures, Cloze techniques, and oral passage-reading measures.

Question answering is the most commonly employed curriculum-based reading comprehension assessment strategy (L. Fuchs, Fuchs, & Maxwell, 1988). However, despite its prevalence, question answering has been subject to several forms of criticism. First, question answering appears to tap comprehension of only selected portions of reading material that have been judged critical by others (Hansen, 1979). Second, correct question answering is related strongly to the passage dependency of questions or the degree to which answers can be inferred directly from questions (Hansen, 1979). Third, systematic methods of generating questions that consistently result in similar reading placements for individual students have yet to be designed (Peterson, Greenlaw, & Tierney, 1978). However, in research comparing the criterion, construct, and concurrent validity of alternative CBM monitoring strategies, L. Fuchs et al. (1988) found that question answering was a viable form of curriculum-based reading comprehension assessment when questions were derived systematically to represent idea units of high thematic importance within passages. Of course, the feasibility of teachers employing such a time-consuming procedure to derive questions for reading comprehension assessment appears problematic.

To monitor reading comprehension through curriculum-based recalls, students read passages from their texts and retell in their own words what occurred in the passages without referring back to text. Recall is a straightforward and feasible CBM strategy in terms of initial preparation. It requires only that suitable reading material be selected. However, methods for scoring recalls can be difficult and time consuming (Johnston, 1982). In investigating alternative CBM reading comprehension measures, L. Fuchs et al. (1988) documented the overall validity of CBM recall methods and compared the validities of alternative recall-scoring methods and production formats. Correlations between criterion outcome measures and total words written during recall, a very feasible scoring procedure, were comparable to more complicated scoring methods. Additionally, correlations with criterion measures were higher for the written production score than for the oral production index. Consequently, a total-words-written retell score may represent a feasible and valid measure for CBM monitoring. To monitor the appropriateness of the recall focus, L. Fuchs et al. (1988) recommended that teachers periodically also score content words retold (i.e., the number of nouns, verbs, adjectives, and adverbs in the retell that match the text).

Cloze is another potential CBM monitoring measure. In typical Cloze procedures, every nth word is omitted from a passage and replaced with a blank. The pupil is required to restore deletions meaningfully. Cloze can be time consuming and expensive to produce: Preparation and photocopy of text with deleted/ underlined words is necessary. On the other hand, scoring methods vary in ease of implementation, with exact replacements a logistically feasible alternative and with synometrically or syntactically correct replacements more difficult. In investigating the acceptability of the Cloze procedure, L. Fuchs et al. (1988) found that written Cloze formats demonstrated adequate criterion and concurrent validity. However, contrary to the other types of CBM reading comprehension measures, the Cloze technique failed to correlate better with reading comprehension than with decoding criterion measures. It is possible that this finding reflects the fact that Cloze may (1) measure textual redundancy rather than comprehension (Tuinman, Blanton, & Gray, 1975), (2) be more dependent on sentence rather than the larger textual context (Suhorsky, 1975), and/or (3) fail to index inferential comprehension and other higher-order reading skills (Alderson, 1978).

A fourth CBM index of reading comprehension is oral reading fluency in which students read aloud under timed conditions while examiners score the number of words read correctly. Tests of oral reading fluency (i.e., the number of words read *correctly* per minute) are (1) easy to prepare, requiring only the selection of appropriate passages and (2) simple to score. Although oral reading fluency traditionally is not viewed as a reading comprehension measure, evidence supports it as an index of reading comprehension (see Chapter 2). Correlations between reading fluency and well-accepted criterion measures of comprehension are consistently strong when (1) both measurements are derived from passages of similar difficulty (Deno et al., 1982; L. Fuchs, 1982a; Gates, 1927) and (2) elementary and/or high school level readers are employed as subjects (Sassenrath, 1972).

Moreover, in comparisons among the validities of question answering, recall, Cloze, and oral reading fluency tests, correlations between all measures and the criterion index of reading comprehension were comparable except one. The oral reading fluency test correlated statistically significantly *higher* with the criterion reading comprehension index than the other measures. Additionally, growth over time on the oral reading fluency CBM monitoring measure has been shown to relate to growth on global tests of reading comprehension (L. Fuchs, Deno, & Mirkin, 1984). Consequently, in the prototypical CBM reading-monitoring system, oral reading fluency is employed as the measurement behavior. That is, teachers regularly measure pupils' oral reading fluency from the goal-level material and employ the resulting data base to formulate decisions concerning the adequacy of student progress in the curriculum over time and the effectiveness of the instructional program in realizing programmatic reading goals.

What Material

As discussed in preceding chapters, an additional dimension for determining "what to measure" concerns the decision over what materials: (1) short-term or mastery measurement or (2) long-term or performance measurement (Deno & Fuchs, 1987). To review, with performance measurement, an annual goal is specified, and a large pool of related measurement items is created. For example, 75 fourth-grade reading passages can be selected as the set of measurement samples. From this measurement pool, monitoring probes are drawn randomly, and the difficulty level of the monitoring probes remains fairly constant over the year.

With short-term measurement, a series of objectives corresponding to steps within a hierarchical curriculum is specified, and a series of small item pools are created, each of which corresponds to a specific objective. The difficulty level of material on which students are measured increases as students master the sequential objectives, and mastery of objectives across time is graphed.

Both types of measurement are ongoing, criterion referenced, curriculum based, and consistent with programmatic goals. However, these systems are conceptually and technically different. With short-term measurement, assessment corresponds more closely to instruction, because the monitoring probes are drawn from the instructional material. For example, if the r-controlled phonics rule were introduced instructionally, the short-term monitoring measure would be reading a list of r-controlled words. By contrast, the long-term monitoring probe might involve oral reading fluency on passages randomly selected from the basal reader.

Although short-term measurement relates better to the current instructional focus, long-term measurement possesses at least two advantages. First, it better represents components of the ultimate desired performance (i.e., reading passages with many types of words fluently). Second, its correlation with global achievement tests, including reading comprehension measures, is stronger than that of mastery measurement (L. Fuchs, 1982a).

Short-term and long-term measurement also have different practical implications. Short-term measurement is easier to understand, and teachers seem to prefer it for communicating progress to other professionals and parents (L. Fuchs, Wesson, Tindal, Mirkin, & Deno, 1982). However, it also can require additional time commitments from the teacher to create new monitoring measures as students master the hierarchy of objectives.

Additionally, differences in student achievement outcomes are associated with these monitoring procedures. In a meta-analysis, L. Fuchs and D. Fuchs (1986b) coded 18 studies in terms of short-term or long-term measurement and in terms of a dependent measure—a probe-like (e.g., reading CVC word lists) or global achievement (e.g., Stanford Achievement Test) test. Results suggested an interaction among these variables. When long-term measurement was used, effect magnitudes on global achievement tests were larger; when short-term measurement was used, effect magnitudes on probe-like measures were greater. Therefore, in developing the prototypical CBM monitoring system, long-term measurement is incorporated. Nevertheless, in certain circumstances, such as for students with minimal incoming skills when it may be difficult to elicit behavior on long-term goal tasks, practitioners may wish to consider short-term measurement.

HOW TO MEASURE

Once the behavior and material to be monitored have been selected, a second task is to specify the mechanics of measurement. Within the decision-making matrix (see Table 6.1), such methodological issues are subsumed under the "how to measure" question and concern measurement duration, frequency, and methods of administration and scoring.

Duration

Duration refers to the length of each curriculum-based test. In considering the effects of duration on technical characteristics of the measurement, L. Fuchs, Tindal, and Deno (1984) demonstrated that correlations between 30- and 60-second curriculum-based reading tests were comparable. To supplement this finding, L. Fuchs, Tindal, and Deno (1984) compared 30-second to 3-minute sample lengths within a multiple-baseline reversal design with two second-grade reading-disabled pupils. The median number of words correct per minute was consistently higher in the 30-second than in the 3-minute presentations with each pupil. Despite the higher estimates of student reading skill levels in the 30-second phases, the corresponding trends over time were relatively flat. In contrast, the trends in the 3-minute phases demonstrated greater increases. Additionally, indices of the variability in the time series indicated lower intraindividual variability and increased reliability with the longer sample duration.

With respect to the effects of sample duration on student achievement outcomes, evidence for the strong relationship between time engaged in appropriate practice activity and student achievement may support the position that student achievement gains observed with CBM monitoring are a function, at least in part, of increased time on task on reading activities associated with measurement activities. If this is so, then as the measurement sample becomes longer, student achievement may improve. However, as described above, results conflict concerning the relationship between the level and slope of performance with alternative sample durations. This finding makes it difficult to establish the instructional superiority of one sample duration.

The logistics consideration relevant to sample duration is readily apparent; that is, the shorter the sample duration, the more feasible the measurement system becomes for teachers to use. In the previously described analyses, sample duration appeared to have no consistent effect on measurement, but longer sample durations did reduce variability. With respect to time on task, one can postulate the instructional superiority of longer samples; yet, no empirical work supports this speculation. Logistically, the shorter durations clearly are preferable. Yet, the difference between 30- and 60-second samples may be practically unimportant in a teacher's schedule: The same cannot be said for 1- versus 3-minute samples. Although definitive recommendations concerning sample duration cannot be drawn from the current data base, a conservative position appears to be one of compromise. Therefore, in designing the prototypical measurement system, we recommend oral fluency samples of 1-minute duration. They are longer than the 30-second sample and therefore allow for some effects on technical characteristics and student achievement to accrue. Moreover, they are one third as long as the 3-minute samples and therefore facilitate the feasibility of the CBM monitoring procedures.

Measurement Frequency

Measurement frequency refers to the number of times per week practitioners measure pupil performance. In terms of technical considerations, White (1972) established that a minimum of seven data points are necessary to project a reliable performance trend. So to ensure an adequate data base on which to support instructional decisions concerning the efficacy of student programs and to avoid prolonged use of inappropriate instructional strategies, practitioners should collect data frequently—ideally, on a daily basis. Additionally, as demonstrated by L. Fuchs, Deno, and Marston (1983), for initially imprecise curriculum-based single measurements of academic proficiency, aggregating estimates of performance over occasions increases the stability of achievement estimates to well within acceptable levels.

Although technical considerations seem to support daily measurement, practical considerations suggest a leaner data collection schedule. Preparing for measurement, measuring, scoring performance, recording scores, and putting away materials can be time consuming. As indicated by logistics research, after field practice with the CBM monitoring procedures, teachers devote over 2 minutes total time per individual reading assessment (L. Fuchs, Fuchs, Hamlett, & Hasselbring, 1987; Wesson, Fuchs, Tindal, Mirkin, & Deno, 1986). Multiplied across a caseload of 15 to 25 students, each of whom is measured in additional curriculum areas, the time teachers devote to measurement can be substantial.

Besides the practical requirement of a less-than-daily measurement schedule, research indicates no additional benefits accruing to student achievement as a function of increasing measurement frequency beyond twice weekly. In a quantitative synthesis of relevant, controlled studies, L. Fuchs and D. Fuchs (1986a) found that the average effect magnitudes associated with measurement that occurs twice weekly, three times weekly, and daily, respectively, were 0.85, 0.41, and 0.69. No significant differences existed among the measurement frequencies.

Current evidence therefore suggests that daily measurement may generate the most technically adequate data base. Nevertheless, practitioners' time contraints mitigate against daily measurement, and student achievement effects associated with daily and twice-weekly measurement appear comparable. Therefore, in building the prototypical CBM monitoring system, we recommend that special education practitioners measure pupils' oral reading fluency for 1 minute twice each week. Twice-weekly measurement allows teachers to collect seven data points in approximately 1 month, allowing sufficient time for (1) demonstration of instructional effects and (2) modification of ineffective programs.

Methods of Administration and Scoring

Over the course of years of working with teachers in implementing CBM monitoring systems and of experimenting with alternative test administration and scoring procedures, Deno and colleagues (see Deno, 1985) outlined oral reading fluency test administration and scoring methods that demonstrate strong technical adequacy, are associated with positive student achievement outcomes, and appear to be feasible for teachers to use. (The reader is referred to L. Fuchs, 1982a, for a discussion of some of this literature.) These procedures are listed in the Appendix for reading as well as for math, spelling, and written expression.

HOW TO USE DATA

Research indicates that teachers who measure student performance data do not necessarily employ the information to evaluate the effects of their instruction (Baldwin, 1976; White, 1974). Therefore, systematic methods for analyzing those data may be critical to effective CBM monitoring systems. In a meta-analysis, L. Fuchs and D. Fuchs (1986a) found that the effectiveness of CBM monitoring was enhanced when teachers used a systematic data utilization strategy. For that reason, careful attention needs to be devoted to how CBM monitoring data are recorded and evaluated.

Recording

The manner in which CBM monitoring data are recorded appears to be critical. Specifically, it appears that graphing rather than simply recording student scores in tabular form relates to positive student outcomes, with student achievement improving approximately 0.5 of a standard deviation unit (L. Fuchs & Fuchs, 1986a) above the effects of ongoing monitoring with recording alone. Additionally, the type of graphing convention may affect student gains.

One type of graphing paper is ratio, where the rate scale is adjusted to display proportional changes in student behavior (White & Haring, 1980). Some propose that this ratio-scaled paper is technically superior (see, for example, White & Haring, 1980) because the ratio scale may reflect the proportional way in which natural change occurs more accurately than equal-interval paper. Also, ratio-scaled paper may be more feasible than equal-interval paper because it displays a larger behavior range.

On the other hand, the second type of paper, conventional equal-interval charts, may facilitate data analysis (see Tawney & Gast, 1984) and be easier for practitioners and parents to understand. Additionally, Marston (in press) explored the prediction capabilities of the two graphing papers and found that, when CBM data are graphed, trend lines on equal-interval paper predicted future performance more accurately than trend lines drawn on ratio-scaled paper.

Despite discussion of the relative advantages of the two types of graph paper, only one contrast of the extent to which graphing conventions influence student achievement is available. L. Fuchs and D. Fuchs (1987b) found that the papers were comparable, with no statistically or practically significant difference between effect magnitudes associated with the types of charts.

Given the lack of clear support for the technical or effectiveness superiority of one type of paper, we include conventional equal-interval paper in our prototypical CBM monitoring system. In CBM field sites, the use of equal-interval chart is standard. Typically, charts display 36–38 weeks of data to reflect one academic year. The primary consideration in formulating this decision has been practical: Teachers and students report that they find the conventional paper easier to understand and read, rendering the CBM monitoring procedures more feasible and usable within classrooms.

Data Evaluation

Research supports the use of data evaluation rules rather than unsystematic teacher inspection of CBM monitoring data for formulation of decisions concerning the adequacy of instructional programs. For example, L. Fuchs and D. Fuchs (1986a) found that, on average, CBM monitoring that incorporated data utilization rules was associated with increased student achievement of approximately 0.5 of a standard deviation unit over CBM monitoring without systematic rules. With rules, the mean effect magnitude was 0.91.

Examples of data evaluation rules are found in the work of Haring, White, and Liberty (1979). These rules require teachers to assess patterns in successive student performance data points in relation to an aimline (or the expected rate of progress), which connects the baseline data with the goal date and performance criterion. These rules (see White & Haring, 1980) are prescriptive; They suggest both when and how to modify programs. Experiments suggest that these rules may increase student outcomes; however, it is unclear whether rules for specifying both when and how to change programs are superior to rules indicating when to change programs (Martin, 1980).

Deno and colleagues have employed "goal-oriented" and "treatment-oriented" data evaluation rules. The goal-oriented approach (see Figure 6.1) is referenced to the aimline: When student performance trends are less steep than the aimline and fall below the expected rate of progress, programmatic modifications are introduced. This approach appears to be conceptually easy for teachers because it is rooted within a traditional,

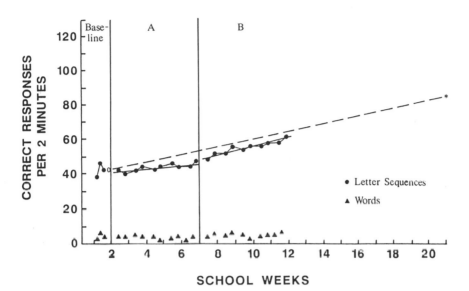

FIGURE 6.1. Example of a goal-oriented data analysis graph.

educational, goal-oriented paradigm (see L. Fuchs, 1988, for discussion)

With the treatment-oriented approach (see Figure 6.2), the effectiveness of the current instructional program is evaluated by comparing it to performance in preceding instructional phases. Instructional changes are introduced at regular intervals. Lines of best fit through actual data points, within different phases, are compared to assess the relative effectiveness of alternative instructional phases. Effective programs are developed cumulatively over time by maintaining useful components and eliminating less effective instructional dimensions.

Research comparing the value of these different data evaluation rules is scarce. In one experimental study, L. Fuchs (1988) found that goal-oriented evaluation may relate to better teacher compliance with rules and with superior student achievement outcomes. Yet, within this study, the use of computers seemed to mediate the effects of the decision rule (see L. Fuchs, 1988, for discussion).

Consequently, although it remains clear that the use of data evaluation rules produces better outcomes than informal inspection of student performance data, a definitive data base support-

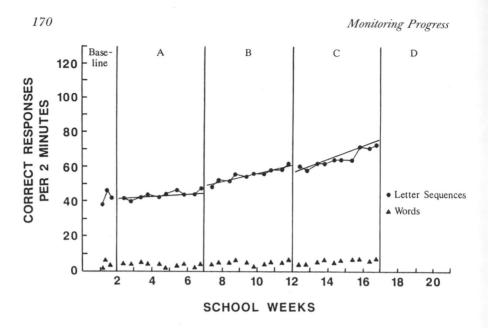

FIGURE 6.2. Example of a treatment-oriented data analysis graph.

ing one type of evaluation system does not exist. In the protypical CBM monitoring system, we recommend the goal-oriented rule for the following reason. Teachers appear to understand and require less training and practice with the goal-oriented data evaluation rule (L. Fuchs et al., 1982). Additionally, the goal-oriented rule appears to produce more reliable decisions than the use of the treatment-oriented data evaluation procedure (L. Fuchs, 1982b). The use of this goal-oriented rule, as well as the application of each of the recommendations outlined above, is illustrated with the case study described below. In CBM field sites, both types of data evaluation are employed.

CASE STUDY ILLUSTRATING THE CBM MONITORING PROTOTYPE

Figure 6.3 displays Darrell's CBM monitoring data over the course of part of an academic year. This CBM graph is a document from which Darrell's reading instructional program can be explained. In reviewing this program, the decision-making steps formulated by Darrell's teacher, Ms. B, are described.

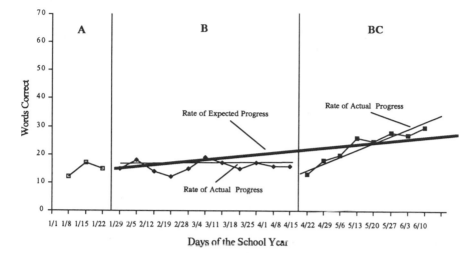

FIGURE 6.3. Example of the CBM graph with correct words read per minute on vertical axis and time, marked in week intervals, on the horizontal axis.

What to Measure

To establish what to measure, Ms. B followed the guidelines reviewed and, therefore, decided to monitor Darrell's oral reading fluency performance. Additionally, Ms. B had to determine the level of material from which she would draw the reading passage stimulus material. Ms. B decided to employ a performance measurement system. Since Darrell's IEP objective had been written using the "expert judgment" procedure described in Chapter 5, the difficulty of the measurement stimulus material represented the level specified in that IEP: grade level 5 of Ginn 720. Darrell's current instructional level was grade level 4 from Ginn 720. However, because of the importance of measuring student improvement on the long-term outcome performance desired at the year's end within performance measurement, Ms. B decided to draw the reading passages for measurement from grade level 5.

How to Measure

Now that Ms. B had determined that she would measure Darrell's oral reading fluency performance in grade level 5 during this academic year, her next step in specifying the CBM monitoring system was to decide how to measure. Once she outlined the mechanics of measurement, these methodological specifications would remain constant across the year. Only with constant measurement conditions can CBM monitoring data indicate student growth rather than reflect modifications in measurement.

Following the guidelines reviewed, Ms. B determined that twice each week she would have Darrell read aloud from a randomly drawn passage from grade level 5 of Ginn 720 for 1 minute, and she would follow the administration and scoring procedures provided. Ms. B began data collection in order to estimate Darrell's initial performance level in grade level 5. The first day's assessment was available from the survey level assessment data used to determine Darrell's eligibility for special education. Over additional school days, Ms. B collected measurement samples as required. On the baseline measurement days, Darrell scored 12, 16, and 14 words correct and 8, 10, and 10 errors. Calculating a median across the data points, Ms. B summarized Darrell's initial, or baseline, performance level in grade level 5 as 14 words correct and 10 errors. As specified in the IEP, to be proficient in grade level 5 by the year's end, Darrell needed to read 70 words correctly with no more than seven errors. This performance level represented Darrell's reading goal, and Ms. B continued to measure Darrell's oral passage reading rate performance in grade level 5, using the same measurement methods, twice each week over the course of the year.

How to Use Data

In accordance with the guidelines reviewed, Ms. B decided to graph Darrell's student performance data on equal-interval paper. The graph in Figure 6.3 displays Darrell's progress over time, as indexed by the CBM monitoring system. The horizontal axis represents school weeks; the vertical axis is the number of words read aloud correctly per minute from grade level 5 of Ginn 720. The first three data points show Darrell's baseline measurements. The beginning point of the heavy solid line indicates the intersection of the median baseline performance with the first day of instructional programming in reading; this introduction of reading instruction also is noted with the first vertical line. Darrell's goal on the graph is represented by the end of the broken line at the intersection of the goal date and the criterion performance level of 70 words correct per minute. The heavy solid line represents the rate at which Darrell must progress in order to attain his goal.

Now that Ms. B was ready to begin the formal reading instructional program, she specified exactly what the nature of that program was, using the five-component instructional plan sheet (see Figure 6.4). Every school day, Ms. B had Darrell read orally for 5 minutes, read silently for 10 minutes, and write and discuss individually with the teacher his recall of the silent reading passage (see intervention labeled B on Figure 6.3). She implemented this program, as specified, for 5 school weeks as she employed the CBM monitoring system. At the end of 5 weeks, when she had collected 10 measurement points, she analyzed the data using the goal-oriented rule described above. As shown with the lighter, shorter solid trend line through Darrell's performance points during intervention B, Darrell's actual rate of progress through this 5-week period was less than expected (see the heavy solid aimline). Therefore, using the goal-oriented approach to data analysis, Ms. B projected that Darrell would not reach his goal if the current instructional program were maintained as is. Ms. B then introduced an instructional modification signified by the second intervention line.

This second intervention represents the introduction of intervention BC (see Figure 6.3). Intervention BC (see Figure 6.4 for description) incorporated every dimension of intervention B, as indicated by the label, but introduced an additional component. Ms. B had Darrell review an instructional schema for organizing his recall each day during the individual session in which they reviewed Darrell's recall. Ms. B implemented this intervention for 3 additional school weeks, concurrent with CBM data collection. At the end of this time period, as indicated on Figure 6.3, Darrell's rate of progress had improved; the slope of the second lighter, shorter trend line was steeper than that of the heavy solid aimline. Ms. B concluded that Darrell would master the goal if he continued to improve in the same fashion. So Ms. B continued to implement intervention BC and continued to measure and reanalyze the data regularly.

The CBM monitoring data allowed Ms. B to evaluate the effectiveness of the reading instructional program systematically. With the CBM data base, she could formatively evaluate and empirically develop an effective program for Darrell. This teaching–testing approach increased the probability that Darrell

INSTRUCTIONAL PROCEDURES PLAN SHEET
Teacher Name: Ms. B.

Student Name: Darrell

Academic Area: Reading

Instructional Procedures	Arrangement	Time	Materials	Motivational Strategies
B				
Oral reading practice	1–1 with teacher	5 min	Level 5, Ginn 720	5 min free time for sat-
Silent read- ing practice	Independent	10 min	Level 5, Ginn 720	isfactory completion
Write recall	Independent	10 min	Silent read- ing passage	of all ac- tivities
Discussion of recall	1–1 with teacher	5 min	Silent read- ing passage	
BC				
Continue as above	1–1 with teacher	Add 5 min to discus- sion of recall activity	Silent read- ing passage	

ADD: Use story map to review recall during discussion of recall

FIGURE 6.4. Example of an Instructional Plan Sheet.

would reach the instructional goal. In a similar fashion, by using key indicators of academic progress, students' programs can be individually tailored in spelling, math, and written expression to permit teachers to improve their instructional pedagogy and decision making and to facilitate improved student achievement.

FUTURE DIRECTIONS FOR CBM MONITORING

Research on CBM monitoring continues. As with any developing system, new applications and varying components constantly are under investigation. For example, current research addresses the potential of peer measurement, the accuracy of alternative methods of drawing lines of best fit, and the appropriate level of difficulty on which to monitor pupil programs. In this section, three developing directions for CBM monitoring are discussed in greater detail: (1) computer applications to CBM, (2) alternative measurement systems, and (3) a modified decision rule.

Computer Applications

In recent years, L. Fuchs, Hamlett, and D. Fuchs (1988) and Germann (1987) have developed software applications for CBM monitoring. L. Fuchs and associates have conducted research to assess the effects of such applications. The rationale for developing such software is threefold: (1) to ensure standardization of the CBM monitoring, (2) to increase the feasibility of the monitoring systems, and (3) to extend the information teachers can derive from the measurement. A description of the computer applications follows; for information on the research and additional information on the software, readers are encouraged to write the author.

The L. Fuchs, Hamlett, and Fuchs (1988) computer applications to CBM involve three basic components: probe generation software, automatic data collection software, and data management software. First, software has been developed to generate CBM assessment materials and to save to disk those probes for monitoring progress in math, spelling, and reading. Answer keys also are saved to disk to allow for automatic scoring of student performance. In math, a set of 81 computation problem types was derived to represent the Tennessee Basic Skills First curriculum objectives (TBSF). The TBSF is a statewide curriculum that is (1) to be mastered by all elementary-age students and (2) assessed by annual criterion-referenced testing. A program then was developed to allow the practitioners to specify up to 25 types of problems to appear on the probe, the number of problems of each type, and the number of pages per probe. The problem order and the numbers within problems are generated randomly by the computer. As stated, answer keys also are generated.

In spelling, the probe generation software creates lists of 20 words randomly selected from a master file of spelling words for the relevant grade level of the spelling curriculum. In reading, software generates reading passage recall probes, which use files of 400-word passages by level of the appropriate reading curriculum. These passages were created using a standard word-processing program. Once information about the appropriate level of reading passages has been entered into the computer, the software randomly samples passages from the appropriate level, from which the pupil reads before recalling information.

The second type of software, which automatically collects student performance data, is called the "Checkups" disk. The Checkups disk contains the automatic data collection software and performance data files for up to eight students in three academic areas. The disk also stores answer keys for the math, spelling, and reading probes for automatic scoring of student performance. Each student also is given a disk of reading passages (called the "Stories" disk) and a folder containing 50 printed spelling lists and 50 math probes. With the data collection disk, CBM monitoring data are collected automatically as the student interacts with the computer. The performance is scored by the computer, and performance feedback, in the form of the student's graph, is provided to the pupil. Student scores and responses are automatically stored for the teacher to inspect at a convenient time with the data management disk.

The third type of software involves teachers' data management. The data management disk (DMD) retrieves, charts, and analyzes student performance data saved on the Checkups disk. The teacher boots up the DMD and identifies the student(s) and academic area(s) for which he or she will review pupil data. The computer than displays a chart for each pupil and each academic area selected. These graphs display (1) data points, (2) aimline, (3) vertical intervention lines to signify the introduction of programmatic changes, (4) a trend line, which shows the pupil's actual rate of progress within the most recent instructional program and which is extrapolated to show the projected proficiency level by the goal date, and (5) graphic and verbal information concerning whether the teacher should make an instructional change to effect better academic growth or raise the student's goal. The teacher can choose to print each graph. Additionally, the teacher can access a summary of the pupil's performance on the probes and receive qualitative feedback concerning the pupil's error patterns. In the area of spelling, for example, the teacher is provided with lists of spelling categories in which the student has made errors, the list of correct spellings, and the list of the student's corresponding errors. Then, the software provides teaching rules for each category, along with an instructional strategy.

This software has the potential to free teachers from the time-consuming tasks of preparing probes, administering tests, and scoring, graphing, and analyzing data. Additionally, consistency in measurement across days is enhanced, and the amount and quality of information teachers receive is increased. Initial research (L. Fuchs & Fuchs, 1987a) indicates that with automatic data collection, teachers save significant and substantial amounts of time in collecting, storing, graphing, and analyzing student performance data. Teachers' roles change from that of data coordinator and generator to instructional expert who inspects the data base and formulates instructional decisions. Research indicates that no negative effects on student achievement are associated with automatic versus teacher-collected student performance data bases. Current research is examining teachers' use of qualitative feedback as well as alternative computer feedback methods, goal formats, and use of expert systems that make instructional recommendations to practitioners within such computerized CBM monitoring programs.

Alternative CBM Measurement Systems

Additional CBM measures of achievement are under development. An example is the expansion of the reading measurement to include more than oral reading fluency. Motivated by the need to identify a reading measure that would be (1) adaptable for computerized data collection with currently available school hardware and (2) valid, reliable, and sensitive to student growth, L. Fuchs et al. (1988) have explored alternative reading measurement systems. Over the course of the 1986–1987 academic year, 10 special education teachers monitored their pupils' reading growth using a Cloze procedure; 10 special educators tracked their students' reading progress with a recall technique; and 10 special educators served as a control group, using no systematic CBM. Findings indicate that the recall procedure may result in superior achievement to the Cloze measure, and the monitoring with the recall measure appears to result in improved student achievement compared to control groups. A comparison of the recall with the oral passage reading procedure is needed. If one or both appear adequate, teachers may prefer the alternative measure because of the ease associated with computerized data collection and superior face validity as an index of reading comprehension (see L. Fuchs et al., 1988, for discussion).

Modified Decision Rules

To review, the data evaluation rule recommended as part of the prototypic CBM system was termed goal oriented. Using this approach, teachers compare actual rates of student progress against those projected on the basis of IEP goal attainment. During the 1986–1987 school year, L. Fuchs, D. Fuchs, and Hamlett (in press) contrasted this rule with a modified goal-oriented approach in the area of math. This modified goal-oriented rule added one dimension to the standard goal-oriented approach: If students' actual rates of progress, projected out in time to the goal date, indicated that the goal would be mastered or exceeded, teachers were required to increase the goal. From then on, teachers analyzed the adequacy of actual progress rates to the rate required to achieve the new goal. Findings indicated that teachers using this modified decision rule increased goals an average of approximately 0.60 times per pupil, whereas teachers in the standard goal-oriented rule group introduced a mean of 0.05 goal increases per pupil. Moreover, final goals for the modified decision rule were significantly higher than for the standard decision rule. Additionally, students in the modified goal-oriented group achieved significantly more than pupils in control groups, whereas students in the standard goal-oriented group did not. These findings are tentative and need to be replicated in other academic areas and with additional pupils and teachers. Yet, results suggest the potential effectiveness of the modified goal-oriented rule, which encourages teachers to increase goals and to be ambitious in their expectations for handicapped pupils. Additional research exploring this as well as additional modifications in the decision rules currently is underway (L. Fuchs, Fuchs, & Hamlett, 1988).

REFERENCES

Alderson, J. C. (1978). Cloze procedures. In O. K. Buros (Ed.), *The eighth mental measurements yearbook* (pp. 1171–1174). Highland Park, NJ: Gryphon Press.

Baldwin, V. (1976). Curriculum concerns. In M. A. Thomas (Ed.), *Hey, don't forget about me* (pp. 64–73). Reston, VA: Council for Exceptional Children.

Deno, S. L. (1985). Curriculum-based measurement: The emerging alternative. *Exceptional Children, 52,* 219–232.

Deno, S. L. (1986). Formative evaluation of individual student programs: A new role for school psychologists. *School Psychology Review, 15,* 358–382.

Deno, S. L., & Fuchs, L. S. (1987). Developing curriculum-based measurement systems for data-based special education problem solving. *Focus on Exceptional Children, 19*(8), 1–16.

Deno, S. L., Mirkin, P. K., & Chiang, B. (1982). Identifying valid measures of reading. *Exceptional Children, 49,* 36–45.

Eubanks, E. E., & Levine, D. U. (1983). A first look at effective schools projects in New York City and Milwaukee. *Phi Delta Kappa, 64,* 697–702.

Fuchs, D., & Fuchs, L. S. (1986). Test procedure bias: A meta-analysis of examiner familiarity. *Review of Educational Research, 56,* 243–262.

Fuchs, D., Fuchs, L. S., Power, M. A., & Dailey, A. (1985). Bias in the assessment of handicapped children. *American Educational Research Journal, 52,* 63–71.

Fuchs, L. S. (1982a). Reading. In P. K. Mirkin, L. S. Fuchs, & S. L. Deno (Eds.), *Considerations for designing a continuous evaluation system: An integrative review* (Monograph No. 20; pp. 29–74). Minneapolis: University of Minnesota Institute for Research on Learning Disabilities.

Fuchs, L. S. (1982b). Data analysis. In P. K. Mirkin, L. S. Fuchs, & S. L. Deno (Eds.), *Considerations for designing a continuous evaluation system: An integrative review* (Monograph No. 20; pp. 116–126). Minneapolis: University of Minnesota Institute for Research on Learning Disabilities.

Fuchs, L. S. (1988). Effects of computer-managed instruction on teachers' implementation of systematic monitoring programs and student achievement. *Journal of Educational Research, 81,* 294–304.

Fuchs, L. S., Deno, S. L., & Marston, D. (1983). Improving the reliability of curriculum-based measures of academic skills for psychoeducational decision making. *Diagnostique, 8,* 135–149.

Fuchs, L. S., Deno, S. L., & Mirkin, P. K. (1984). Effects of frequent curriculum-based measurement and evaluation on pedagogy, student achievement, and student awareness of learning. *American Educational Research Journal, 21,* 449–460.

Fuchs, L. S., & Fuchs, D. (1986a). Effects of systematic formative evaluation on student achievement: A meta-analysis. *Exceptional Children, 53,* 199–208.

Fuchs, L. S., & Fuchs, D. (1986b). Curriculum-based assessment of progress toward long- and short-term goals. *Journal of Special Education, 20,* 69–82.

Fuchs, L. S., & Fuchs, D. (1987a). *Improving data-based instruction through computer technology: Continuation application.* Unpublished manuscript available from L. S. Fuchs, Box 328, Peabody College, Vanderbilt University, Nashville, TN 37203.

Fuchs, L. S., & Fuchs, D. (1987b). The relation between methods of graphing student performance data and achievement: A meta-analysis. *Journal of Special Education Technology, 8*(3), 5–13.

Fuchs, L. S., & Fuchs, D. (1987c). *Effects of curriculum-based measurement procedures in spelling and math.* Unpublished manuscript available from L. S. Fuchs, Box 328, Peabody College, Vanderbilt University, Nashville, TN 37203.

Fuchs, L. S., Fuchs, D., & Butterworth, J. (in press). Effects of curriculum-based measurement on student awareness of learning. *Education and Treatment of Children.*

Fuchs, L. S., Fuchs, D., & Hamlett, C. L. (1988). *Effects of alternative data-evaluation rules within curriculum-based measurement.* (Research Report No. 416). Nashville, TN: Peabody College of Vanderbilt University.

Fuchs, L. S., Fuchs, D., & Hamlett, C. L. (in press). Effects of alternative goal structures within curriculum-based measurement. *Exceptional Children.*

Fuchs, L. S., Fuchs, D., Hamlett, C. L., & Hasselbring, T. S. (1987). Using computers with curriculum-based progress monitoring: Effects on teacher efficiency and satisfaction. *Journal of Special Education Technology, 8*(4), 14–27.

Fuchs, L. S., Fuchs, D., & Maxwell, L. (1988). The validity of informal reading comprehension measures. *Remedial and Special Education, 9*(2), 20–28.

Fuchs, L. S., Fuchs, D., & Stecker, P. M. (in press). The effects of curriculum-based measurement on teachers' instructional planning. *Journal of Learning Disabilities.*

Fuchs, L. S., Hamlett, C. L., & Fuchs, D. (1988). *Improving data-based instruction through computer technology: Description of Year 3 software.* Available from L. S. Fuchs, Box 328, Peabody College, Vanderbilt University, Nashville, TN 37203.

Fuchs, L. S., Tindal, G., & Deno, S. L. (1984). Methodological issues in curriculum-based reading assessment. *Diagnostique, 8,* 19–26.

Gates, A. I. (1927). An experimental and statistical study of reading and reading tests. *Journal of Educational Psychology, 12,* 303–313, 378–391, 445–464.

Germann, G. (1987). *Pine County Special Education Co-op Software.* Sandstone, MN: Author.

Gersten, R., Carnine, D., & White, W. A. T. (1984). The pursuit of clarity: Direct instruction and applied behavior analysis. In W. L. Heward, T. E. Heron, D. S. Hill, & J. Trap-Porter (Eds.), *Focus on behavior analysis in education* (pp. 38–57). Columbus, OH: Merrill.

Goodman, L. (1985). The effective schools movement and special education. *Teaching Exceptional Children, 17,* 102–105.

Hansen, C. L. M. (1979). Chicken soup and other forms of comprehension. In J. E. Button, T. Lovitt, & T. D. Rowland (Eds.). *Communications research in learning disabilities and mental retardation.* Baltimore: University Park Press.

Haring, N. G., White, O. R., & Liberty, K. A. (1979). *Field initiated research studies: An investigation of learning and instructional hierarchies in severely and profoundly handicapped children: Annual Report 1978–1979.* Seattle: University of Washington, Child Development and Mental Retardation Center, Experimental Education Unit.

Hoffman, J. V., & Rutherford, W. L. (1984). Effective reading programs: A critical review of outlier studies. *Reading Research Quarterly, 20,* 79–92.

Johnston, P. B. (1982). *Implications of basic research for the assessment of reading comprehension* (Research Report No. 206). Urbana-Champaign: Center for the Study of Reading. (ERIC Document Reproduction Service No. ED 201 987)

Lloyd, J. W. (1984). How should we individualize—Or should we? *Remedial and Special Education, 5,* 7–15.

Marston, D. (in press). Measuring academic progress of students with learning difficulties: A comparison of the semi-logarithmic chart and equal interval paper. *Exceptional Children.*

Martin, M. A. (1980). *A comparison of variations in data utilization procedures on the reading performance of mildly handicapped students.* Unpublished doctoral dissertation, University of Washington, Seattle.

Peterson, D. L., Albert, S. C., Foxworth, A. M., Cox, L. S., & Tilley, B. K. (1985). Effective schools for all students: Current efforts and directions. *Teaching Exceptional Children, 17,* 106–111.

Peterson, J., Greenlaw, M. J., & Tierney, R. J. (1978). Assessing instructional placement with the IRI: The effectiveness of comprehension questions. *Journal of Educational Research, 71,* 247–250.

Rieth, J. H., Polsgrove, L., & Semmel, M. I. (1981). Instructional variables that make a difference: Attention to task and beyond. *Exceptional Education Quarterly, 2*(3), 61–72.

Salvia, J., & Ysseldyke, J. E. (1985). *Assessment in special and remedial education.* Boston: Houghton-Mifflin.

Sassenrath, J. M. (1972). Alpha factor analyses of reading measures at the elementary, secondary, and college levels. *Journal of Reading Behavior, 5,* 304–315.

Snow, R. E., & Lohman, D. F. (1984). Toward a theory of cognitive aptitude for learning from instruction. *Journal of Educational Psychology, 76,* 347–376.

Suhorsky, J. (1975). *An investigation of the relationship between undeleted text preceding a Cloze test and Cloze test results.* Unpublished doctoral dissertation, University of Maryland, College Park.

Tawney, J. W., & Gast, D. L. (1984) *Single subject research in special education.* Columbus, OH: Merrill.

Tuinman, J. J., Blanton, W. E., & Gray, G. (1975). A note on Cloze as a measure of comprehension. *Journal of Psychology, 90,* 159–162.

Wesson, C., Fuchs, L. S., Tindal, G., Mirkin, P. K., & Deno, S. L. (1986). Facilitating the efficiency of ongoing curriculum-based measurement. *Teacher Education and Special Education, 9,* 84–88.

White, O. R. (1972). *Methods of data analysis in intensive designs.* Paper presented at the annual meeting of the American Educational Research Association.

White, O. R. (1974). *Evaluating educational process* (working paper). Seattle: University of Washington, Child Development and Mental Retardation Center, Experimental Education Unit.

White, O. R., & Haring, N. G. (1980). *Exceptional teaching* (2nd ed.). Columbus, OH: Merrill.

Ysseldyke, J. E. (1979). Psychoeducational assessment and decision making. In J. E. Ysseldyke & P. K. Mirkin (Eds.), *Proceedings of the Minnesota Roundtable Conference on Assessment of Learning Disabled Children* (Monograph No. 8). Minneapolis: University of Minnesota, Institute for Research on Learning Disabilities. (ERIC Document Reproduction Service No. ED 185 765)

7

Periodic and Annual Reviews and Decisions to Terminate Special Education Services

Donald Allen

The previous chapters have discussed how CBM provides a data base for making each of the psychoeducational decisions regarding a student's educational program; it also provides a continuous data base that indicates how a student is performing in the curricular material being taught in the classroom. The purpose of this chapter is to present CBM procedures for conducting periodic and annual reviews so that decisions about the effectiveness of any special education program can be made. Norm-referenced and idiographic comparison procedures are detailed to determine the benefits of classroom instruction. Special emphasis is given to procedures for making decisions to exit a student from special education.

When CBM measures are normed on the local population of students, they provide a valuable reference for making screening decisions. By comparing a student's performance on grade-level material to that of his or her peers, it is possible to identify which students are far enough behind to warrant further assessment of their academic needs. Prior to referral, collecting continuous data on the student using CBM makes it possible to evaluate the relative effectiveness of the prereferral interventions. Once referral for special education programs is deemed appropriate, these measures are also very useful in determining eligibility for service. By testing across grade-level materials, information can be collected to determine if additional services are warranted (i.e., a special education program) to redress the skill deficiency. By closely monitoring students' responses to specific instructional strategies, one can gather important information regarding specific instructional and placement needs. The formative evaluation approach utilized with CBM allows for identification of effective instructional strategies via direct and efficient evaluation of student progress.

One important set of decisions that is made with handicapped students has not yet been addressed, however, that of periodic and annual reviews. Periodic reviews usually take place informally on a per-grading-period basis (e.g., quarterly, by trimester). Annual reviews occur at the expiration of the individual education plan (IEP). The purposes of these decision-making activities are twofold: (1) to determine if the intervention activities specified in the IEP are sufficient or need adjustment and (2) based on this determination, to decide whether a major change in instructional program and/or level of service is required. Whereas the notion of change in instructional program is straightforward, the proposition of change in level of service is more complex. The question is related directly to a decision by the multidisciplinary team (MDT) that a change in level or placement, either to a more or less restrictive setting, is required for a student. Such decisions include the termination or exit of a student from special education and return to the regular education classroom on a full-time basis. It is interesting that while eligibility decisions for special education services are viewed as the major concern and responsibility for the school psychologist (Reschly, 1982; Shinn, 1986), the decisions made at periodic and annual reviews typically do not involve school psychologists, nor are they discussed frequently in school psychology or special education texts or literature. The topic of change in level of service, including exit from special education, receives attention only indirectly through discussion of special education effectiveness (Marston & Magnusson, 1988; Shinn, 1986).

CURRENT STATUS OF ANNUAL REVIEWS AND EXITING HANDICAPPED STUDENTS

The rules and regulations for PL 94-142 (Section 121a.552) require that "Each public agency shall insure that: (a) Each handicapped child's educational placement: (1) Is determined at least annually." This regulation constitutes the legal requirement for the annual review. Unfortunately, specific procedures to be used to determine if a special education program is effective and/or a change in level of service is required are not detailed in the rules and regulations for implementing PL 94-142. Based on an examination of the special education literature, little assistance is available. Negligible importance is given to the procedures for conducting this process. This conclusion is supported in a study of the special education identification and decision-making procedures in use across the United States by Chalfant (1984). He observed that although states typically include pages of procedures for identifying, evaluating, and placing students in special education ". . . only a few paragraphs or pages concern the transition of students into declining levels of services or how to dismiss students from services which are no longer needed" (Chalfant, 1984). McNutt (1986) reported that only a few states include any information on exit criteria, and Gartner and Lipsky (1987) reported considerable frustration in their efforts to obtain information from Federal sources on the topic. They provided this quote from a letter they received from the U.S. Department of Education in response to their efforts to obtain exit data.

> Thank you for your letter in which you ask about data concerning children who have been certified as handicapped and have returned to regular education. While these are certainly very interesting data you request, these data are not required in state plans nor has the office of Special Education Programs collected them in any other survey.
>
> [Letter to Alan Gartner from Patricia J. Guard, Deputy Director, Office of Special Education Programs, U.S. Department of Education, November 7, 1986 (Gartner & Lipsky, 1987, p. 367).]

It may be that data typically are not collected on students' exist from special education because it is not a very common event. When data do exist, they reinforce this suspicion. Gartner and Lipsky (1987) reported that in their sample of 26 large cities, fewer than 5% of the students in special education return to general education annually. The decision to make a change in level of service, from a more restrictive placement to exit, based on an evaluation of special education's effectiveness is a crucial decision and should not be ignored or treated as trivial. Another viable hypothesis is that the data collected, if any are collected systematically, are insufficient to allow this decision to be made reliably.

A CONCEPTUAL MODEL OF PERIODIC AND ANNUAL REVIEW

In the business world, there is a common understanding that the best way to begin a partnership is with rules on how to dissolve that partnership. It would bode well for school psychologists and special educators to adopt this concept to special education decision making. Thus, any discussion of exit decisions must be linked to discussion of eligibility.

When a student is referred for special education services, it must be determined if the student is (1) eligible for and (2) in need of service in special education (Bateman & Herr, 1981). Even after the student is placed in a special education program, eligibility and need remain issues. Need remains an issue primarily because we aspire to reach a point with that student that it becomes necessary to ask the question if the student is still in need of special education assistance. Need and eligibility for mildly handicapping conditions such as learning disabilities are related clearly to the magnitude of discrepancy between the handicapped student and the achievement expectations of the regular classroom (see Chapter 4). This discrepancy is operationalized as a level difference between the achievement of the handicapped student and peers at the point of placement, as demonstrated in Figure 7.1.

Decision-making procedures for making changes in level of service, including exit, are needed for students whose instructional needs change over time. The premise behind special education services is that providing special instruction to handicapped students can reduce the discrepancy between how the student is performing relative to peers over time. As indicated in Figure 7.1, the expectations of the regular classroom are changing as the typical achievement of peers increases over time. The achievement gains of any particular handicapped student are unknown and are represented in Figure 7.1 by lines A, B, and C. The academic gains made by a student relative to the regular education expectations determine how effective and appropriate special education help is. As discrepancies between special education students and their peers are reduced (as indicated by line A), at the time of the periodic or annual review, it may be necessary to discontinue special education service and/or place the student in a less restrictive special education environment. If the difference in level remains constant (as indicated by line B), a decision may be made to maintain the status quo, change the intervention, or make a change in level of service. If the discrepancy between the special

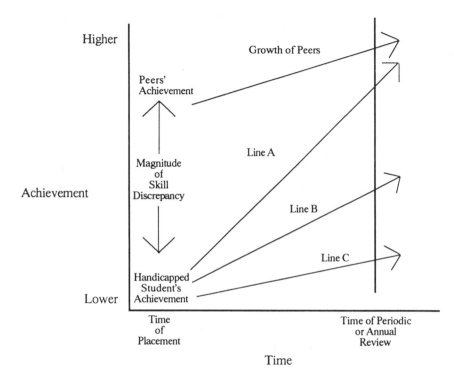

FIGURE 7.1. A conceptual model of evaluating achievement changes of a handicapped student relative to the growth of peers.

education student and peers increases (line C), then it may be necessary to consider the possibility of a change in the level or type of service.

Thus, it is clear that eligibility for service remains an issue after initial placement because of the possibility that the student may no longer be eligible for or in need of service if a less restrictive program is appropriate or if the intervention provided is ineffective and the student requires a different program.

CONDITIONS FOR EXITING STUDENTS FROM SPECIAL EDUCATION

The decision to terminate students from special education is a special form of change-in-level decision that is made during periodic or annual reviews. Because of its importance, it warrants special consideration. Two major reasons prevail as to why an MDT might consider a child no longer eligible for special education service. These reasons are simply the reverse of the two conditions that were met when the student was initially placed in special education: (1) the child might no longer be handicapped, or (2) the child might no longer be in need of service. For example in the case of a learning-disabled student two conditions must be met. First, there must be a discrepancy between what the child has learned and what was taught. "If there is no severe discrepancy between what should have been learned and what has been learned, there would not be a disability in learning" (Federal Register, 1977b). It is assumed that what is taught is what should have been learned. Second, there must be no apparent reason other than a learning disability why this discrepancy exists. In essence, this mildly handicapping condition, this learning disability, is defined by default. No other reason can be found for the child's failure.

Although it is made quite clear that these two conditions result in placement in special education, it is not stated clearly that students are removed from service when these conditions no longer exist. Instead, it is stated only generally in PL 94-142 that MDTs must assess and evaluate handicapped children's programs on a regular basis to determine if placement is appropriate (i.e., that the programs are effective and that the students remain eligible). It is only assumed that students are monitored and assessed to determine if they are still handicapped and in need of service.

RIGHT PROCESS—WRONG DATA BASE

In a study of how states implement the provisions of PL 94-142, Chalfant (1984) addressed the issue of annual review. In spite of the lack of specific procedures and criteria in Federal and state law, Chalfant found that there was a considerable amount of agreement among states as to what conceptual issues should be addressed in the annual review process. The results from a questionnaire on assessment and identification procedures suggested that presence of a handicap and need for service are the issues that must be attended to. Specifically, Chalfant found three specific assessment questions that were frequently mentioned.

1. What are the expectations for the student in the current instructional setting (i.e., special education) as well as in any new setting (i.e., more or less restrictive) that is being considered?
2. What is the nature of the student's academic, social, emotional, or physical needs (strengths and weaknesses)?
3. Is the student benefiting from the intervention, and will he/she continue to benefit?

Together these three questions form a rational basis for evaluating the effectiveness of an individual's special education program and for making decisions regarding change in level of service. It seems, then, that even though specific procedures and criteria for conducting periodic reviews are not prescribed, schools are attempting to focus on the appropriate issues. Given a legal requirement for the periodic and annual review process and a solid rational basis that focuses on the appropriate evaluative issues, why is it that the decision-making process receives so little attention in practice? One likely explanation is that the assessment data collected are insufficient to address the three questions asked earlier. That is, the information collected during students' periodic and annual reviews is not relevant or is not collected with sufficient frequency to answer the previous questions.

Determining the Expectations

Critical components that are implied in the question about expectations in the instructional setting are knowledge of the goals of (1) the instructional intervention and (2) any other placement setting being considered. Goals for the former are to be found in the short-term and long-term goals of the IEP. Goals for the latter are based implicitly on the levels of academic achievement for the setting being considered. For example, for a change to less a restrictive placement (i.e., the regular education classroom), knowledge of the expectations of student performance (i.e., the typical peers) provides a critical standard for decision making.

As detailed in Chapter 5, typical goals for IEPs are particularly problematic, as the objectives are either too general or too specific for evaluative purposes. It seems likely that little valid decision making can occur with respect to the expectations of the special education program if the goals are poorly written. Objective assessment of the expectations of any other placement setting is also problematic as quantitative data too often are unavailable. This paucity of data reflects the field's preoccupation with assessing only students and not environments. Rather than assessing environmental expectations, most typically, expectations are based on estimates of a student's "potential" as measured by intelligence tests. Students with higher scores are expected to accomplish more from an instructional intervention than those students with lower scores. This "prediction orientation" has been characterized as problematic (Reschly, Kicklighter, & McKee, 1988c), and little if any data exist to suggest how intelligence tests can be used to operationalize expectations for individual evaluations of student progress.

CBM offers an obvious advantage for identifying the expectations for students' IEPs and for those alternative placement settings. The components of the IEPs written with CBM reflect the specific curriculum level in which the student is expected to perform as well as an expected criterion for the IEP to be considered successful. For example, an annual goal from an IEP is written similar to "In 36 weeks, when given a randomly selected passage from Reading Mastery Level D, the student will read aloud 100 words correctly with 5 or fewer errors." The expectations are explicit.

Determining Needs

A student's need is operationalized as a difference in level between what is expected and a student's current abilities or aptitudes. At the point of eligibility, traditionally, the most common ability that is assessed is the student's general intellectual ability. The results of these ability assessments are presumed to help to identify specific disabilities and are used to measure an expected achievement–achievement discrepancy. It is on this determination that many students are placed in special educational programs.

The relevance of this operationalization of need has been questioned (Reschly, Kicklighter, & McKee, 1988a, b, c). In a series of decisions, the courts have ruled that students must only be grouped academically according to some educationally relevant variable. Ability tests only measure a correlate of academic performance, and student performance on these measures is affected by many educationally irrelevant factors. As a result, placement in special education programs based on these measures does not necessarily reflect actual educational need.

Interestingly, a shift in how need is measured occurs once a student is placed in special education. Currently, every 3 years, the "need" that qualified a student as handicapped is reassessed using similar methods. Once in a program, assessment of need shifts typically to pre–post testing on published achievement tests. This strategy, at best, is useful only for determining the effectiveness of the intervention. As a result, it could be argued that one of the primary purposes for annual reviews, to examine a student's needs, is ignored.

One potential solution would be to measure ability–achievement discrepancies on a pre and post basis. However, proponents of CBM decision making would argue that, instead, need should be operationalized directly and assessed continually. Initial special education placement based on direct measures of student achievement in the curriculum being taught reflects educational need. In reviewing the decisions of the courts in several important cases, Reschly et al. (1988a) concluded that "A grouping plan based primarily on direct measures of skills in an agreed upon curriculum was therefore much easier to defend." Further, any assessment of the effectiveness of the intervention program contributes directly and immediately to conclusions about the handicapped student's current need for special education. Reschly et al. (1988a) emphasized this point, suggesting that ". . . CBA and other direct measures of functioning are preferable because the results are related to interventions beneficial to the individual."

Determining Instructional Benefit to Student

The final question addressed in the periodic and annual process is whether the student is benefiting from the special education intervention that is provided. This issue should be related, in part, to the results of the assessment of the student's needs discussed above. That is, a portion of the determination of benefit is based on a determination of the level of student skills relative to a prescribed set(s) of expectations.

As detailed in Figure 7.1, a special education program is considered beneficial if growth is seen on the variable identified earlier as a weakness for that student. Typically, the results of pre- and posttesting on published, norm-referenced achievement tests (usually at the beginning and end of the school year) are compared to see if any gain or growth is seen. Unfortunately, many of the measures typically used for this purpose are inappropriate for evaluating student achievement (Jenkins & Pany, 1978; Good & Salvia, 1987) and thus inappropriate for determining the effectiveness of the instruction provided. These measures are often insensitive to the specific objectives of the curricular material and insensitive to small amounts of growth over a short period of time. Demonstration that a measure is sensitive to student growth is a technical adequacy issue that generally is not addressed (Carver, 1974) by test developers. For more information on this topic, the reader is referred to Chapter 2.

In contrast, CBM's content validity and sensitivity to the effects of short-term intervention are well documented (Deno, 1985, 1986; Marston & Magnusson, 1985, 1988). Decision making can be accomplished using CBM to assess idiographic change relative to the expectations expressed in the IEP and normative change relative to the achievement expectations for students in other settings.

PROCEDURES FOR USING CBM FOR PERIODIC AND ANNUAL REVIEW DECISION MAKING

It is necessary to describe what CBM data to collect and discuss specific guidelines as to how to use these data to make decisions.

It was argued earlier that periodic and annual review are designed to answer the following questions:

1. Are the intervention activities specified in the IEP sufficient for the student to progress according to the designated expectations or do they need adjustment?
2. Based on the answer to 1, is a major change in instructional program and/or level of service required?

Procedurally, the assessment activities for periodic and annual reviews are similar. What varies between the two undertakings is that, generally, the assessment activities at the annual review are more thorough, and a formal written report is required.

Assessing Benefit

As stated above, assessing the benefit of the special education program to the handicapped student is the primary purpose of the periodic and annual review. This process is accomplished according to two approaches: idiographic and norm-referenced.

Ideally, the first idiographic strategy for determining benefit would be to compare students' rates of academic progress without and with special education services. To accomplish this task, it is necessary to compare the student's slope of improvement before placement in special education to the trend of improvement after placement in special education. If the student's trend of improvement is greater when in special education than when receiving instruction in the regular education program, then special education intervention would be considered to be beneficial. This conclusion could be true even if normative evaluation suggested no reduction in the student's discrepancy from typical grade-level peers. The fact remains that the student learned at a faster rate when receiving special education assistance. It could be concluded that special education placement provided a more efficient instructional strategy than the mainstream classroom.

This is the case illustrated in Figure 7.2. In this example, Mary was placed in special education because her performance was significantly below that of her grade-level peers in written expression. It is obvious from the CBM data that the regular education intervention was not appropriate for Mary because her rate of improvement was significantly lower than that of her peers. She was falling further behind. After she was placed in special education, her rate of improvement climbed significantly. Mary was learning at a faster rate in her special education program. Even though Mary may have failed to decrease the skill difference from her peers, it could be argued that special education service was beneficial and that the intervention program should be maintained.

It should be pointed out that these data usually are not available for assessing the benefit of special education programs for individual students. Most frequently, the determination of benefit demands that a formal examination of the student's progress towards the IEP objective take place. Using the goal-oriented treatment approach described in Chapter 6, the slope and level of student achievement are compared to the expected rate of improvement stated in the IEP goals. When a periodic review is conducted, the criterion for success is a level of student performance that approximates an intersection of the student's line of expected progress on their graph and the date of the review. An example is presented in Figure 7.3.

At the time of the first periodic review (1/1), Ann was expected to be performing at a rate of about 38 words read correctly per

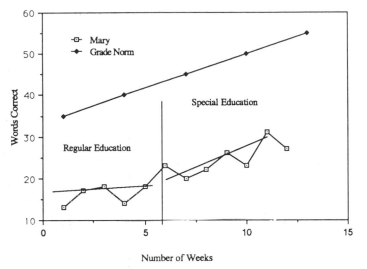

FIGURE 7.2. A comparison of Mary's progress in written expression in regular and special education intervention programs relative to the progress of her peer group.

minute. Her actual performance was 45 words. Thus, it could be concluded that at that time, her instructional program in special education was beneficial.

When an annual review is conducted, the student's level of improvement must approximate that specified by the criterion in the IEP objective. For example, in Figure 7.3, Ann was expected to read 75 words correctly by the time of the annual review (5/1). Because she read only about 50 words correctly, according to the goal-oriented treatment approach it could be concluded that her program had not been as beneficial as projected.

A second strategy for evaluating the benefit of special education is to use the treatment-oriented approach detailed in Chapter 6. The slope of improvement under the most recent instructional program is compared to the slopes obtained during special education interventions attempted earlier during the school year. If student trend has not improved significantly since that first intervention, then the special education service possibly is not beneficial. As exemplified in Figure 7.3, at the time of the annual review (5/1), it could be concluded that although Ann had not met the IEP long-range goal of 75 words per minute, trend line C suggests that her current intervention is more beneficial than the instruction represented by trend line B.

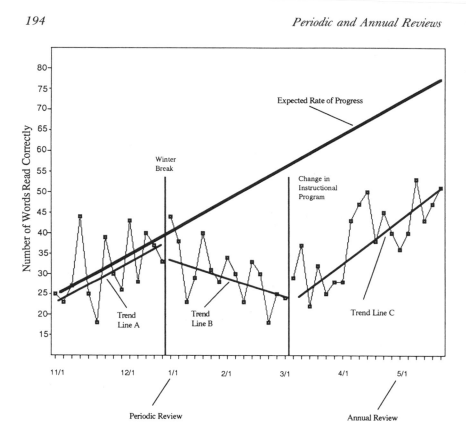

FIGURE 7.3. The use of a goal-oriented treatment approach for evaluating the effectiveness of special education programming.

Normative CBM data also are useful in determining benefit. Again, change in performance is the critical variable. However, instead of comparing students to themselves, a comparison is made of change in student performance relative to expectations (i.e., a normative sample). For a periodic review, the procedures employed during CBM screening are repeated. Students are tested on grade-level materials at the time the norms were developed, and their scores are compared to the normative sample. Several different standards can be applied to determine if the amount of student gain was sufficient to indicate that special education service was beneficial. First of all, the standards typically employed with any pre–post evaluative model can be used. The type of metric (e.g., discrepancy scores, standard scores) can have differential effects when student growth is assessed (Tindal, Shinn, & Germann, 1987). The use of change in discrepancy scores is problematic, as they are not equal-interval data. Whereas discrepancy scores can be used to determine gross change (i.e., positive relative growth, negative relative growth), for more exact estimates of growth, changes in standard scores are recommended. These scores can be converted to percentile ranks for communication purposes. An intervention is determined to be beneficial if the student reduces the difference in level of skill from grade-level peers.

For annual reviews, the process more closely approximates those procedures used to determine a student's eligibility. Students are tested not only on grade-level materials from their academic areas listed on the IEP but also on curriculum materials at levels of typical students in grades below. Sample results from an annual review of a special education student's testing in reading are presented in Table 7.1.

On entry into special education, the student performed below the first percentile of grade-level peers and below the fourth percentile of students one grade below. Evaluative strategies similar to the periodic review are used to interpret these normative data. In this example, by the time of the annual review, the student had improved relative to the peer group, to the second percentile of same-grade peers and to the 10th percentile relative to students one grade below. It is likely that the MDT would consider special education beneficial for this student.

By integrating the data obtained from the idiographic and normative approaches, MDTs can fully evaluate the effects of special education for individual students. Each combination of

TABLE 7.1. A Comparison of Handicapped Student's Median Reading Scores and Percentile Ranks in Different Grade-Level Materials at the Time of Entry into Special Education and the Annual Review

Grade level material	Student's entry raw score	Student's annual raw score	Student's entry percentile rank	Student's annual percentile rank
4	43	59	<1	2
3	54	67	4	10
2	58	89	15	23
1	70	115	69	95

outcomes from each approach has different implications. Insufficient growth on both types of measures would suggest that, at the very least, the instructional program be modified. If students reached their IEP objective at the time of their annual review but growth relative to the norm was less than was desired by the MDT, it suggests that their IEP objectives were insufficiently ambitious. A potential change in making the expectations of the instructional programs more challenging could be considered. Other decision-making ramifications of different outcomes are presented in Table 7.2.

Assessing Need

Earlier, it was discussed how CBM procedures could be used to determine the degree of benefit of special education for handicapped students. The question of need remains. Clearly, the concepts of benefit and need are closely related. If the intervention was determined to be nonbeneficial, then the issue of student need becomes moot. If a CBM system has been employed to monitor student progress, it is likely that several intervention changes have been noted and implemented already. At the time of the annual review, it might be quite possible to make a strong recommendation regarding a change in the level of service provided and to consider the environmental demands of any alternative program.

If benefit can be shown (i.e., if student trend has improved and

TABLE 7.2. A Comparison of Potential Outcomes from Idiographic and Normative Evaluation Strategies and Their Ramifications for Periodic and Annual Review Decision Making

Growth relative to IEP objective	Growth relative to normative sample	Decision-making ramification
No	No	Ineffective program. Change instructional program.
Yes	Yes	Effective program. Consider need.
Yes	No	Program effects uncertain. May be unambitious goals.
No	Yes	Program may be effective. Goals may be too ambitious.

relative standing has changed positively), it then becomes more complicated to determine student needs. Does the student need less service, if any at all, or should the same service be provided? Under these circumstances, it is highly desirable that strong consideration be given to instruction in a less restrictive environment. In these instances, attention must focus less on relative levels of performance and more on absolute levels of skills. That is, can the handicapped student perform at some level of skill in the curriculum that will maintain him/her in the alternative setting?

Determining When to Exit

In instances when termination of special education services is being considered, it is necessary to decide if the student's level of performance is adequate relative to the demands being placed on students in the mainstream classroom. Peer skill levels define the least restrictive environment (LRE). The most logical operationalization of LRE is that of the immediate classroom to which the student would be returned. Two potential comparison groups are available. Most typically, students are considered to be mainstreamable if their performance falls within the average range of performance of their grade-level peers (i.e., within one standard deviation of the mean for their grade level). This perspective is quite controversial (Marston, 1988), since "within the range of grade-level performance" may prove to be too strict a standard for mainstreaming.

Marston (1988) offered a different comparison standard that perhaps reflects a more realistic concept of LRE. He argues that often when students are returned to the mainstream, they are not expected to compete with the average peer. Instead, they may be accepted in the classroom if they can perform within the expectations for other lower-performing students (Gerber & Semmel, 1984). Special education students need only be able to compete with the students in the lowest instructional group.

An alternative procedure in such a case would be to compare the student's performance level to the mean performance level of the low-curriculum group. With the simplicity of administration of the CBM measures, it is quite easy for the teacher to collect monthly norms on the low-curriculum group to serve as a standard. When the student performs above the median performance level of the low instructional group, the child may be ready to return to the mainstream via the low instructional group. Consider, for example, John's performance in math as presented in Figure 7.4.

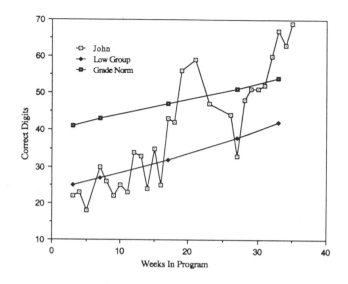

FIGURE 7.4. A comparison of John's performance in math to the mean performance of the low curriculum group and the grade-level norm.

In this example, CBM procedures were used to determine John's performance level in math and the performance expectations in a less restrictive environment, regular education. The broken line in the figure represents John's performance on CBM in math each week. As indicated in the graph, John improved steadily since he had been placed in the special education program. By assessing a sample of students in the regular education environment, his MDT was able to establish performance expectations for both average grade-level performance and desired performance in the lowest regular education math instructional group in that school. In the graph, the upper straight line reflects mean performance in math for students in John's grade in his school. The lower straight line reflects the mean performance level of students in the low math group at John's grade level. The low instructional group provides the first opportunity for John to return to the mainstream and serves as an appropriate standard for determining when John might be ready for exit from special education. In this example, John was placed in the low regular education curriculum group after week 30, when his performance in math was consistently above the mean of that group.

No hard and fast rules have been tested empirically about when a less restrictive environment or a lower level of service might be appropriate. The decision to change level of service initially must be a decision made by the MDT and must represent their collective opinion as to what is appropriate for any particular student. The appropriateness of the level of service ultimately decided on can only be determined *post hoc* by collecting student progress data systematically. If the child's trend of improvement increases in rate or remains at or near the rate seen during special education, then the decision regarding level was appropriate.

SUMMARY

There is no reason to assume that student needs or adequacy of intervention changes only on a 1-year cycle. The assessment time-lines described in PL 94-142 provide minimal standards, not the most desirable or efficient condition. Placement or level-of-service issues must be considered from the initial day of placement to time of exit and beyond. The CBM procedures allow for viable and efficient decision making regarding the effectiveness of special education and continued need, including level of service, during a student's periodic and annual reviews. The effectiveness of the special education intervention is determined by comparing student progress towards the IEP objective and academic gains relative to the normative sample. Taken together, these methods can contribute to conclusions regarding student need. Decisions regarding exit from special education can be made in the context of operationalizing the level of student skills necessary to fit into existing instructional groups in the regular classroom. When students are considered for termination, their rates of progress in levels of the curriculum used in the regular education classroom can be assessed and compared to the skills of other students at that instructional level. When the performance of the handicapped student is in the range of other students consistently, it appears logical that the student should be terminated from special education.

We must be careful to monitor student progress past the time of exit to determine if the exit decision was correct. CBM is unique in that it provides a measurement approach that makes exit or change in level a continual issue. Exit is linked to entrance as well as to monitoring of the effectiveness of instructional strategy. A common metric and decision-making model is used, and these issues can be addressed continually during the time the child is receiving service. In this way, changes in service or program can be made according to student need rather than according to an arbitrary assessment schedule.

ACKNOWLEDGMENT

The author wishes to thank W. David Tilly for his work on the figures for this chapter. He is a doctoral student in school psychology at the University of Oregon.

REFERENCES

Bateman, B., & Herr, C. (1981). Law and special education. In J. M. Kauffman & D. P. Hallahan (Eds.), *Handbook of special education* (pp. 330–360). Englewood Cliffs, NJ: Prentice-Hall.

Carver, R. P. (1974). Two dimensions of a test: Psychometric and edumetric. *American Psychologist, 29,* 512–518.

Chalfant, J. C. (1984). *Identifying learning disabled students: Guidelines or decision making.* Burlington, VT: Northeast Regional Resource Center, Trinity College.

Deno, S. L. (1985). Curriculum-based measurement: The emerging alternative. *Exceptional Children, 52,* 219–232.

Deno, S. L. (1986). Formative evaluation of individual programs: A new role for school psychologists. *School Psychology Review, 15,* 358–374.

Federal Register (1977a) Regulations implementing Education for All Handicapped Children Act of 1975 (Public Law 94–142). *Federal Register,* August 23, *42*(163), 42474–42518.

Federal Register (1977b). Procedures for evaluating specific learning disabilities. *Federal Register,* August 23, *42*(163), 65082–65085.

Gartner, A., & Lipsky, D. K. (1987). Beyond special education: Toward a quality system for all students. *Harvard Educational Review, 57,* 367–395.

Gerber, M., & Semmel, M. (1984). Teachers as imperfect tests: Reconceptualizing the referral process. *Educational Psychologist, 19,* 137–148.

Good, R. H., & Salvia, J. (1987). Curriculum bias in published, norm-referenced reading tests: Demonstrable effects. *School Psychology Review, 17,* 51–60.

Jenkins, J. R., & Pany, D. (1978). Standardized achievement tests: How useful for special education? *Exceptional Children, 44,* 448–453.

Marston, D. (1988). The effectivenss of special education: A time-series analysis of reading performance in regular and special education settings. *The Journal of Special Education, 21,* 13–26.

Marston, D., & Magnusson, D. (1985). Implementing curriculum-based measurement in special and regular education settings. *Exceptional Children, 52,* 266–276.

Marston, D., & Magnusson, D. (1988). Curriculum-based assessment: District level implementation. In J. Graden, J. Zins, & M. Curtis (Eds.), *Alternative educational delivery systems: Enhancing instructional options for all students* (pp. 137–172). Kent, OH: National Association of School Psychologists.

McNutt, G. (1986). The status of learning disabilities in the states: Consensus or controversy? *Journal of Learning Disabilities, 19,* 12–16.

Reschly, D. J. (1982). Assessing mild retardation: The influence of adaptive behavior, sociocultural status, and prospects for nonbiased assessment. In C. Reynolds & T. Gutkin (Eds.), *The handbook of school psychology* (pp. 209–242). New York: John Wiley & Sons.

Reschly, D. J., Kicklighter, R., & McKee, P. (1988a). Recent placement litigation, Part I, Regular education grouping: Comparison of Marshall (1984, 1985) and Hobson (1967, 1969). *School Psychology Review, 17,* 9–21.

Reschly, D. J., Kicklighter, R., & McKee, P. (1988b). Recent placement litigation, Part II, Minority EMR overrepresentation: Comparison of Larry P. (1979, 1984, 1986) with Marshall (1984, 1985) and S-1 (1986). *School Psychology Review, 17,* 22–49.

Reschly, D. J., Kicklighter, R., & McKee, P. (1988c). Recent placement litigation, Part III, Analysis of differences in Larry P., Marshall, and S-1 and implications for future practices. *School Psychology Review, 17,* 39–50.

Shinn, M. R. (1986). Does anyone care what happens after the refer–test–place sequence: The systematic evaluation of special education program effectiveness. *School Psychology Review, 15,* 49–58.

Tindal, G. A., Shinn, M. R., & Germann, G. (1987). The effect of different metrics on interpretations of change in program evaluation. *Remedial and Special Education, 8,* 19–28.

8

Evaluating the Effectiveness of Educational Programs at the Systems Level Using Curriculum-Based Measurement

Gerald Tindal

The purpose of this chapter is to show how curriculum-based measurement (CBM) can be used in program evaluation. Borich and Nance's (1987) definition of the evaluation process serves as a foundation: "information about the effectiveness of a program, product, or procedure." Three areas must be considered in special education: (1) compliance, maintaining consistencies with local, state, and Federal guidelines and policies; (2) coordination, maintaining an integrated organizational and service delivery model; and (3) changing programs and/or documenting their outcomes. Of the latter two, "The focus areas of coordination and behavioral change should be included in any model to specifically address issues related to program efficiency and student and staff growth" (Borich and Nance, 1987).

Based on the Borich–Nance model, two components are detailed: (1) determination of the worth or merit of a program relative to alternatives and (2) examination of effectiveness based on program outcomes. Therefore, although many evaluation tenets are employed, emphasis is given to output analysis in currently existing programs. This chapter focuses on outcome measurement of interventions for existing programs rather than on program components (Stake, 1976; Stufflebeam et al., 1971) or more systematic and scientific designs that have appeared in the research literature (Fitz-Gibbons & Morris, 1978). As Gersten and Hauser (1984) note, the purpose of evaluation is "to assess whether a change in student outcomes is due to the set of specified variables (in our case usually an educational program) or to other, unexplained factors."

For this chapter, a program is considered a planned and multi-component intervention taking place over an extended period of time and delivered by one or more professionals with a goal of improving student performance. This definition is very similar to Maher and Barbrack's (1979) description of a special service program:

> An organized configuration of program staff (e.g., school psychologists, speech therapists) engaged in programmatic activities (e.g., counseling, language development) using a particular amount of resources (e.g., money, materials) over a set time interval (e.g., daily, weekly) in order to assist one or more pupils to attain certain program goals (e.g., improved self understanding, increased skill in verbal communication) (p. 414).

The chapter is confined to program evaluation at the systems level, where interventions have been delivered to more than one student. Although Borich and Nance's model (1987) includes a range of service options, including self-contained programs, consultation services, support services, related services, and contracted services, the data on CBM procedures are not that extensive. Thus, the text, tables, and figures represent only one service delivery mode: resource room and partially self-contained services. However, instructional programs are defined broadly as they occur in resource rooms. The common link is that instruction is delivered to one or more students by one or more professionals over an extended period of time in an effort to improve academic or social performance.

THE IMPETUS FOR EVALUATING PROGRAMS

Although instructional programs are delivered to individual students—indeed, a central premise of this volume is on the develop-

ment and evaluation of instructional programs for each student—
it is important to attend to the outcomes of these programs at the
systems level. The major impetus for evaluating programs comes
from the need to (1) report program outcomes, (2) develop an
empirical foundation to support them, and (3) establish stable and
representative program features so that they can be replicated.

Reporting Intervention Outcomes

The primary reason for collecting data at the systems level is to
report intervention effects for many students. As a consequence,
an abundance of information is generated, requiring that outcome
data be reduced to a comprehensible level. Whereas data collection itself is a relatively simple and straightforward task, using the
data to determine the effectiveness of a program is a complex and
often convoluted process. Similar to the considerations reported in
Chapter 5 on monitoring progress toward IEPs, the use of systems-level data to evaluate programs must reflect several important issues: (1) the purpose of evaluation or type of decision to be
made, (2) the audience for whom data are to be presented, and (3)
the type of data to collect and report. At the systems level, with
data coming from many sources, the amount of information must
be reduced systematically and presented in an understandable
fashion.

Developing an Empirical Foundation

Another reason for evaluating programs is to justify their implementation. Systems-level data represent the most sensible and
empirical foundation from which to develop educational programs with demonstrated positive educational effects. Scores are
aggregated to reflect program outcomes for students in general
and can serve as a basis for initiating similar programs with other
students.

Consider two programs, A and B, each deployed with comparable groups of students. Program A is found to result in more
improvement than program B, as evidenced by higher summary
scores. For most students, then, program A should be implemented. However, this outcome does not mean that such a
program is optimal for *all* students. For some individuals, program B may well have been more effective, but in the aggregation
of scores from many individuals, more students in program A
improved than in program B.

Establishing Stable Program Features

The final reason to evaluate programs is to examine external validity, which is established when educational procedures are applied to different students in different settings by different teachers with the same outcomes. Since it is likely that programs differ in implementation across students and teachers over time, aggregation of data provides a generalized and summative view. Instead of concentrating on the effects of an instructional program on one individual on one day, a systems-level program evaluation sums data across individuals and over time. Positive program effects are averaged with less-than-positive effects, and peak-performance days are collapsed with some low-performance days. By averaging all sources of variation, any effects are likely to be more stable and applicable across a range of conditions and individuals. If a particular educational delivery system is employed in a school system, data collected from all implementors can be aggregated to determine overall effects. It is likely that programs are implemented differently across individuals and settings; thus, a range of program interventions occur. If significant effects can be attained with individual variation present, such effects are more trustworthy.

ASSUMPTIONS OF THE EVALUATION PROCESS

Several premises are required before an educational program can be evaluated. The first and most important assumption is that the data base on student performance is reliable and valid. Chapter 2 reviewed much of the literature on the technical adequacy of curriculum-based measures. The second supposition is that the purpose of evaluation is to make a decision for an individual student or a group of students. Third, data inherently reflect a unit of analysis and level of program (individual or various sizes of groups). The fourth postulate is that data must be collected in a manner that is sensitive to the audience, which consists of those who will receive the evaluation report or who actually will make the decisions. These assumptions become relevant in both establishing and conducting evaluations.

APPROACHES TO THE EVALUATION PROCESS

The purpose, audience, and type of data are important in considering the design for evaluating any educational program.

The last issue, determining the type of data to collect, is covered in detail in the rest of the chapter. Specifically, three types of data are considered: norm referenced, criterion referenced, and individual referenced. Each of these dictates a different measurement sampling plan and evaluation design.

In the traditional norm-referenced assessment (NRA), the scores of students in the treatment group are compared to scores of a large norm group of students on the same test (Tallmadge, 1981). To be applicable to such a large group, the tests often are constructed with item difficulty as the major selection criterion. Little consideration is given to matching tests to what is taught in the classroom; therefore, content validity may be suspect.

In a criterion-referenced assessment (CRA), a more specific instructional domain is established for sampling items. Additionally, a systematic procedure is considered in sampling items, and a criterion for determination of mastery is specified (Popham, 1978).

In an individually referenced assessment (IRA), the major criterion for item selection focuses on development of many instructionally relevant alternate test forms to generate a frequent measurement system capable of administration over an extended period of time. In this approach, a student's performance is compared successively to previous levels. The emphasis is on change over time.

The perspective taken in this chapter is that all three approaches are necessary in evaluating educational programs. However, they should be considered in light of the purpose of the evaluation, type of decision, and audience. Whereas NRAs sample from a broad domain, CRAs and IRAs are more related to the content of instruction and allow for more content validity of the test. The criterion-referenced approach is highly related to immediate instructional outcomes, whereas the individual-referenced approach represents more generalizable outcomes.

CONCLUSION AND PERSPECTIVES

In summary, program evaluations must be predicated on a systematically diverse data base that incorporates a wide range of learner outcomes and employs multiple references: norm-, criterion-, and individual-referenced assessments. Such diversity will provide a richer and more comprehensive data base from which to make valid interpretations. In this process, however, we must not lose sight of the major educational interventions or grouping variables that are being evaluated. Programs must be defined in a meaningful manner.

A complete program evaluation also must address delineation of programs—physical arrangements of learning environments, content of curricular materials, and formats of interactive teaching behaviors—without which any evaluation findings are hollow. By focusing on evaluation without simultaneous validation of systematic instructional planning and implementation efforts, we can make no empirical generalizations. But by considering instruction and concurrently measuring outcomes, teachers can develop and implement optimal programs. Nevertheless, this chapter addresses only outcome measurement.

The remainder of this chapter covers NRA, CRA, and IRA as they are applied within CBM. Descriptions of the evaluation strategies come first, followed by parameters, then a review of the empirical support generated for their use. Finally, their deployment within an actual evaluation effort is prescribed.

NORM-REFERENCED ASSESSMENT

As described by Horst, Tallmadge, and Wood (1975), a norm-referenced strategy compares a group of students to a similar group that typically has taken a standardized test at an earlier time. Specifically, a (sub)group of special education students is administered selected CBM at the same time as a (sub)group of regular education students, and the outcomes are compared to determine potential differences, all of which can be reported in a variety of ways. Traditionally, only published tests have been used to evaluate programs, but the same methodology may be adopted with curriculum-based measures.

Summary Metrics and Their Applications

To use CBM in a norm-referenced domain, four components are addressed: (1) determination of testing times, (2) establishment of administration and scoring systems for the CBM measures, (3) analysis of resulting score distributions, and (4) development of reporting formats.

Testing Times

Although most published achievement tests employ fall and/or spring testing times, the majority of school districts using CBM procedures have generated normative data at three times: fall, winter, and spring. As detailed in Chapter 4, fall testing typically is conducted in late September or early October; winter testing is completed in middle to late January; and spring testing is done in late May or early June. An important prerequisite in establishing testing times is to ensure that tests will not be given immediately following a break (i.e., summer or Christmas breaks), since performance may be affected inadvertently because of schedule changes, warm-up on school tasks, attentional conditions, etc.

Another issue is the need for approximately equal intervals in trisecting the school year, which allows for comparable times to look at growth. This consideration is critical for monitoring the normal growth exhibited by regular education students as reflected by the sequence of skills in the curriculum. For example, in the norms generated in Pine County (Tindal, Germann, & Deno, 1983), differential growth between successive norming periods was suspected, since the gain from the fall to the winter was always greater than that attained between the winter and the spring. However, since the time intervals were the same, this effect was more likely a function of the sequence of skills in the curriculum than an artifact of the testing intervals.

Finally, concurrent testing times must be maintained for all students. For a true norm-referenced design, CBM measures must be administered at the same times for both the original norm group and special education students. Differences in the timing of the testing easily can skew the data, invalidating the conclusions of any effects. For example, if the regular education norms were completed in the early fall and special education students were tested in the late fall, performance differences between these groups might be underestimated. Subsequent testing later in the school year (winter and spring) might not reflect true differences in change of the special education students relative to the regular education students.

Administration and Scoring Systems

As covered in the previous chapters on curriculum-based measures, many tasks are available. An important issue in the use of curriculum-based measures in norm-referenced evaluation designs is their sensitivity to change. Deno and associates developed rate-based rather than accuracy measures (Deno, Mirkin, Chiang, & Lowry, 1980; Deno, Mirkin, Lowry, & Kuehnle, 1980;

Deno, Mirkin, & Marston, 1980). Timed tasks were considered less prone to ceiling effects, allowing normal distributions to be established.

Additionally, the scoring metric has a great impact on the measure's sensitivity. As Tindal, Germann, and Deno (1983) reported in an analysis of fourth-grade students in spelling, the distributions are much broader and more bell-shaped with correct letter sequences than with words spelled correctly. Similarly, in reading, the score distributions for word lists and passages are very different, with performance considerably more restricted in the former than the latter.

Distributions of Scores

Since the establishment of local normative samples using CBM in Pine County, districts in various regions of the country have normed their regular education student populations. The resulting data have served as the comparative basis for norm-referenced evaluations. However, in this process, the suitability of the norms as comparison standards must be empirically validated prior to their use in evaluating the effectiveness of other educational programs such as special education.

Analysis of normative data should (1) determine that the norms are distributed normally in an approximate bell-shaped curve except when generally not expected, (e.g., beginning first grade) and (2) derive both measures of central tendency and dispersion. If a plot of the normative data reveals a nonnormal distribution, problems can appear later in the evaluation of outcomes.

In most instances, CBM norms are distributed normally. Sometimes, positively skewed distributions can occur in which most students earn low scores, with only a few scores appearing at the middle and high ends of the scale. This outcome often is present in reading and other academic areas in first grade in the fall because most first-grade students begin their schooling with low skill levels. An opposite problem occurs when many students earn high scores and only a few scores appear at the low end of the scale. This result is typical at the end of the year in spelling, when most students have mastered all the words or when high school students are tested on easy material (i.e., sixth-grade level).

As described earlier, the scoring system for many CBM measures can influence the shape of the distribution. The graphs in Figure 8.1 represent the same group of students whose spelling

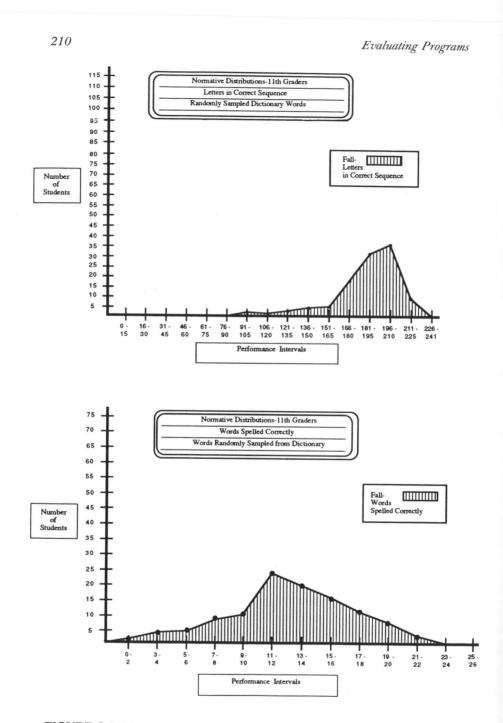

FIGURE 8.1. Normative data from spring performance in spelling: correct letter sequences and words spelled correctly for students in 11th grade.

has been scored in two ways. The bottom graph plots frequencies of students on the number of words spelled correctly. A normal distribution is generated. The top graph, where the number of students whose spelling scores are expressed as correct letter sequences, reflects a negatively skewed distribution. In the normal distribution (words spelled correctly), the students have been spread out consistently; in the latter distribution (correct letter sequences), the students are all at the high end (negatively skewed), a finding often appearing with the use of material that is too easy. In this graph, little distinction can be made among students since they are all so close together in performance. Changes in performance likewise would be difficult to ascertain, since all are so close to the maximum score possible.

These graphs represent findings opposite of those reported by Tindal, Germann, and Deno (1983), in which letters in correct sequence generated a more normal distribution than correctly spelled words. In this earlier study, students were in fourth grade. The students for whom distributions are plotted in Figure 8.1 were in 11th grade. These data suggest that most 11th graders can spell most of the letters in the correct sequence and that only when the entire word is spelled correctly can distinctions be made among the students. By implication, then, scoring systems must be analyzed by their effect on the distribution of scores, with few universalities apparent (i.e., always use the most sensitive scoring technique).

Reporting Formats

The final issue in the use of CBM within a norm-referenced approach is the manner in which data are reported. Two systems generally are employed, incorporating raw scores and percentile ranks or using a graphic plot of the data (frequency polygon), as presented in Figure 8.1.

Given a normal distribution, two summary measures should be calculated: (1) a measure of central tendency (mean or median) and (2) the amount of variation (standard deviation) in the distribution. In some districts, the median has been used to represent the general levels of the norm group. The advantage is that extreme scores are not counted in its calculation, because it represents the score appearing in the middle of the distribution. With half of the scores above and half below, no attention is given to the actual size or values of the scores appearing in the distribution. In other districts, means have been calculated for the norm group, providing a score capable of further manipulation in establishing confidence intervals. Although standard deviations appear complex, this index is useful in representing the amount of variation in the normative population and is particularly helpful in measuring change relative to the general variation present in the population.

As displayed in Figures 8.2 and 8.3, a frequency polygon also can be formatted to communicate data from different grades/normings. In Figure 8.2, data from a math measure given in the spring are displayed across grade levels, with deciles marked off on the y-axis. In Figure 8.3, the distribution has been marked with quartiles. The box represents the 25th to the 75th percentile, and the hatch mark represents the 10th and 90th percentiles (see key).

Issues in the Use of a Norm-Referenced Approach

Assaying the effectiveness of any program using a norm-referenced approach is very complicated, contrary to the elegant but simple description by Glass (1978), who compared students from two groups, one comprised of an experimental status (special education) and the other considered the norm (regular education). Among the more obvious issues in special education evaluation are (1) who should be in the norm group, (2) how should the domain for sampling items be defined, and (3) what is the metric for making comparisons between the groups.

Determining an Appropriate Comparison Standard

The ethnic and demographic composition of the norm group rarely is a problem in CBM because local norms are used. But the constitution of the group as a standard for evaluating change in performance may be an issue. The data presented in the three graphs cited previously have employed regular education students for the normative sample group.

Fuchs, Fuchs, Benowitz, and Berringer (1987) questioned the validity of norm-referenced tests for handicapped students. They noted that such tests often lack a description of the normative sample and fail to provide information on validation of the instruments with handicapped individuals. These issues are equally important in the use of CBM procedures, although a considerable amount of research has appeared in the professional literature

PERCENTILES/RAW SCORES
SPRING NORMING
MATH

NUMBER OF DIGITS
COMPUTED ON
MIXED OPERATIONS

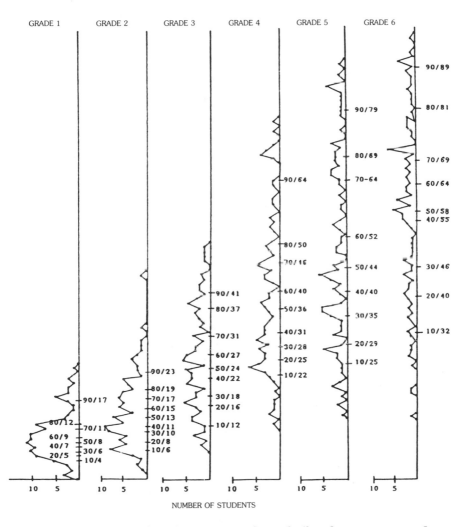

NUMBER OF STUDENTS

FIGURE 8.2. Normative data expressed as deciles for raw scores for elementary students tested in the spring on mixed math operations and scored for digits correct.

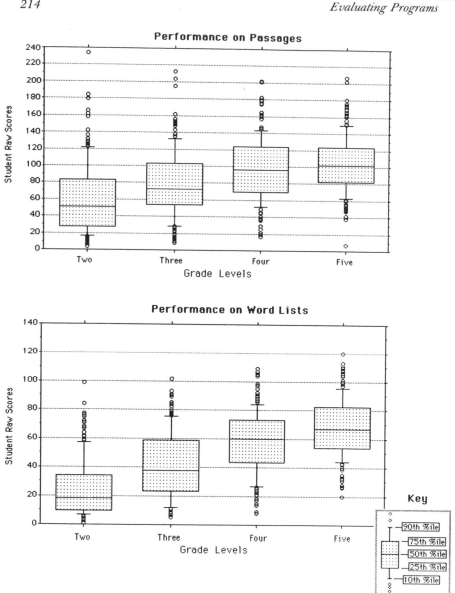

FIGURE 8.3. Normative data expressed in percentile bands for elementary students tested in the fall on two measures of reading: passages and word lists.

that supports its use in a wide range of decisions. Typically, the normative sample includes all students except those served in special education. Most often, the norms are meant to represent the status of regular education only, providing an index from which to mark either a discrepancy or a goal for attainment. Nevertheless, other definitions of normative samples may be appropriate.

The appropriateness of the typical regular education student as a comparison standard may be questionable. The average student in regular education may represent a performance level far greater than that needed by the special education student to be successful in that environment. A more appropriate comparison may be the lowest-performing students in regular education who are nonetheless maintaining minimally successful levels. This group could be comprised of the lowest 50% of students in the regular education classroom, Chapter I students, or students in the lowest skill groups in the regular education classes. The performance levels of these students would then serve as an appropriate comparison group for evaluating special education.

Composition of the CBM Measures

As reviewed in Chapter 4, the manner in which items are sampled for inclusion in norm-referenced tests has a great impact on the data generated. Generally, it is important to (1) maintain a comparable sampling plan over the course of the year, and (2) generate a normal distribution. Both issues focus on test difficulty and/ or the breadth of the domain sampled. Sampling plans that have been used to date most frequently have drawn items from an entire grade. Further coverage of different sampling plans appears in the section on criterion-referenced testing.

Determining the Metric for Summarizing Data

The final issue in evaluating educational programs in general and special education in particular is the reduction of data. In the development of local norms, several metrics are available for representing the average performance of regular education students, including a host of transformed scores. One strategy is to report the average (mean) or median of students in special education at each of the norming periods and compare it to the average or median of the normative sample in a posttest-minus-pretest format, summarizing outcomes in terms of gain. An alternative is to employ a transformed score (e.g., T- or Z-score, discrepancy index, or percentile rank). Again, the two groups are compared within each norming period, and changes in this metric are plotted across successive norming periods.

In Table 8.1, the median performance of students served in special education reading programs in Pine County is reported for successive norming periods—fall, winter, and spring—employing three different metrics. The overall change from the fall to spring norming is shown in the last column. Two transformed scores are calculated for each of these norming periods by comparing special education students' performance to regular education peers: a discrepancy index (Deno & Mirkin, 1977) and a T-score. As explained in Chapter 4, the discrepancy index is calculated by comparing the median performance of each student with the median of the appropriate norm group. The T-score is simply a Z-score with a mean of 50 and a standard deviation of 10. Once all students' performances have been converted to this metric, they are averaged within each norming period.

As can be seen from the values reported in the table, the students in special education were well below their regular education counterparts. On the discrepancy index, they appeared to be well

TABLE 8.1. Outcome Measures for Raw Scores, Discrepancy Index, and T Scores for Each Norming Period in 1983–84 on Reading and Spelling (Correct Letters and Correct Words) Tasks

	Norming period			
	Fall	Winter	Spring	Gain
Reading ($n = 150$)				
Raw scores	22.0	32.0	40.0	18.0
Discrepancy index	−2.9	−2.5	−2.3	0.6
T scores	35.4	35.1	37.4	2.0
Spelling letters ($n = 45$)				
Raw scores	49.0	77.0	102.0	53.0
Discrepancy index	−2.7	−2.2	−2.1	0.6
T scores	31.7	38.0	35.0	6.3
Spelling words ($n = 45$)				
Raw scores	7.0	7.0	11.0	4.0
Discrepancy index	−3.8	−3.3	−2.6	1.2
T scores	28.4	38.0	33.1	4.7

over two times discrepant, with some improvement occurring throughout the year. Their *T*-scores indicated equally low performance, approximately 1.5 standard deviations below the mean of students in regular education norm group.

Although raw scores are simple to calculate, they are very difficult to interpret; because students are from different grades, scores are not directly comparable. Transformed scores (i.e., *Z*-scores, percentile ranks, *T*-scores), however, can be compared over time, setting, and students. This metric takes into account the amount of change or growth in one group (special education) relative to the change or growth in another group (grade-level students from a normative sample). It should be noted that the transformation of scores within each curriculum also makes it possible to collapse data across various curricula, norming periods, and grade levels in reporting them at the systems level. For example, since four curricula were used in the reading programs in Pine County, the raw scores from different programs could not have been compared directly. Therefore, transformed scores were used to provide relative comparisons that are accurate.

Empirical Results on Student Achievement with NRA

Three studies have applied norm-referenced assessments to evaluate special education programs using CBM. Tindal, Germann, Marston, and Deno (1983) analyzed data from students who had been served in resource rooms for the school year in four basic skill areas—reading, math, spelling, and written expression. All CBM measures administered at the beginning, middle, and end of the year were standardized grade-level tasks employing rate of performance as the outcome measure. In the initial determination of eligibility for special education, referred students were compared to a grade-level norm group, and if their performance was two or more times discrepant (Deno & Mirkin, 1977), most were placed in a resource room. Importantly, these students subsequently were reviewed in a periodic (midyear) and annual (end-of-year) evaluation.

The effectiveness data used in the study by Tindal, Germann, Marston, and Deno (1983) were the changes in the discrepancy ratio (i.e., posttest discrepancy scores minus pretest discrepancy scores). The finding was that special education was effective in reducing special education students' average discrepancy from the fall to the spring in reading, spelling, written expression, and math. However, no statistical tests were calculated on the outcomes.

A few years later, Shinn (1986) conducted the same type of evaluation, using much of the same methodology in a different district. He measured students in special education and analyzed their Z-score performance in the fall, winter, and spring. In contrast to the finding by Tindal, Germann, Marston, and Deno (1983), Shinn found that special education was not effective if the purpose was to improve students in special education performance to the levels of their regular education peers. In fact, few students improved in their relative standing over the course of the year. The majority of special education students actually performed at lower levels than their regular education peers over the course of the school year.

Although both studies employed similar methodology by using CBM norm-referenced approaches (similar sampling plans, administration procedures, testing periods, and scoring strategies), two important differences were evident. The former study was completed in a rural educational cooperative, whereas the latter was done in a large urban metropolitan area. Also, the two studies employed different summary metrics; a discrepancy index was used in the former study, and standard scores were employed in the latter study.

In an attempt to reconcile these outcomes, Tindal, Shinn, and Germann (1987) compared several summary metrics using the same population of students from special and regular education. They found that the evaluation metric for summarizing change is an important consideration in determining whether the change is "real" or not: the results were a function of the metrics used. In this study, although gains were evident in the raw scores, no such improvement was evident when special education student performance was summarized with standard scores. Use of the discrepancy index resulted in inconsistent findings; on some measures (reading), special education students showed improvement, whereas on other measures (spelling words correctly), no improvement was shown.

Prescriptions on Using a Norm-Referenced Approach

Three specific issues need to be addressed in completing a norm-referenced evaluation of special education programs involving specification of the type of data to collect, delineation of data collection strategies, and description of procedures for reporting the outcomes.

What Data to Collect

A survey level set of tasks are needed that are grade specific or across grades. Some rationale must exist for selection of the material from which the items are sampled (i.e., modal reading book, range of words or problem types to be presented through a spelling series or math curriculum, or any other range of items to be presented within the evaluation period). A measurement net (more than one single measure or metric) much like that described in Chapter 4 is useful, so that any anomalies in the data can be double-checked across the different measures.

How to Collect the Data

This issue involves the organization of measurement material and administration of the measures. The most efficient strategy for collecting normative data is to use trained volunteers, parents, or school specialists such as resource room teachers and/or Chapter I teachers. These individuals can be trained easily in a half day, and all materials can be sent to each school with one or two teams of two people each. In Pine County, community workers were trained to administer the measures in a 2-hour workshop, assessed for interscorer reliability, which was found to be quite high (from 0.80 to 0.99), and then paired to work in individual schools (Tindal, Germann, & Deno, 1983). In contrast, in Minneapolis, all special education students are typically tested by resource room personnel at the time of the referral. Regardless of who tests the students, the most time-consuming aspect of a norm-referenced curriculum-based evaluation is scoring protocols and summarizing data.

How to Report the Data

Since the premise of a norm-referenced approach is to establish comparable performance levels from a range of students, the two most immediate and practical strategies for reporting scores are percentile ranks and a frequency polygon of raw scores. As displayed in Figures 8.1, 8.2, and 8.3, data from normings can be displayed graphically in many ways. Further graphs employing interpretive guides (either standard deviations or percentile bands) may be useful in making eligibility or mainstreaming decisions.

Summary of Current Status on NRAs in Program Evaluation

A norm-referenced approach to evaluating educational programs encompasses two distinct groups of students, one an experimental group (special education) and the other a standard for making comparisons (regular education). To employ this procedure, it has been noted that group compositions must be appropriate, distributions sensitive, and the outcome metric valid. This approach should be applicable across a range of programs whether the evaluation is of a special education, a reading curriculum, a level of service, or any other grouping of individuals and content.

CRITERION-REFERENCED ASSESSMENTS

In response to the extensive use of norm-referenced evaluations, where broad domains are sampled that are not tied clearly to any instructional focus, increasing emphasis has been placed on a criterion-referenced evaluation strategy. Here, items are drawn from a specified instructional domain. A systematic sampling plan is used and a standard of performance set to determine whether students have mastered the material.

This strategy has been used almost exclusively with the published tests in specific curricular programs and basal series as well as in the establishment of IEP goals and objectives. In the Houghton-Mifflin in Reading Program (Durr, LePere, & Pikulski, 1981), a test of basic reading skills appears at the end of each magazine (a unit of reading material) in Towers—Level H (Brzeinski & Schoephoerster, 1981). These tests sample items from the instructional unit, using a sampling format to ensure that the skills taught are also tested. Typically, a student's performance must be above 80% accuracy within each of a series of subtests (6 to 10 in total) in each magazine. If mastery is attained, the student is allowed to move on to the next unit; if mastery is not attained, instructional review is provided, and the student is retested. Another example of this evaluation format appears in the IEPs of many special education programs. An objective from an IEP might read: "Given a pair of words that have the long vowel sound—some of which are the same and some of which are different—and the direction, 'I am going to say two words, tell me if they are the same,' the student will perform with 100% accuracy."

As both of these examples indicate, three components of criterion-referenced testing must be specified: (1) a well-delineated domain for sampling items, (2) an explicit procedure sampling those items, and (3) a standard of performance for establishing mastery. As reported in Chapter 5, the procedures for CBM do not rely as extensively on this task analytic perspective, in which the curriculum is broken into a sequence of skills. Nevertheless, the establishment of long-range goals and short-term objectives within the IEP does represent a specific domain from which items are generated, a sampling plan is described, and a standard of performance typically is established for determining mastery.

Generally, the learning of individual students is evaluated, and only occasionally has the criterion-referenced approach been used to assay the overall outcomes at the systems level. The following statement may be made when this approach is used at the systems level: "The reading program was successful because 90% of the students passed 80% of the mastery tests with 90% or greater accuracy."

Summary Metrics and Their Applications

The difficulty/discrimination of the item and the standard for mastery must be appropriate for a criterion-referenced evaluation to be meaningful. If a test consists of items that are very easy and/or difficult, any evaluation will be influenced unduly by the fact that many or few students have passed the item. In contrast to the norm-referenced approach, where items of middle-level difficulty are sampled, in a criterion-referenced approach, items are selected according to item discrimination. This index focuses on how discerning an item is in predicting mastery and may be influenced in part by how difficult an item is on the test.

A related issue is the establishment of a meaningful criterion of mastery. Livingston and Zieky (1982) summarized many procedures for establishing mastery, including those proposed by Angoff (1971), Nedelsky (1954), Ebel (1972), and Livingston (1980). These indices of mastery may be interpreted differently; frequently little guidance is provided for selecting among them. Even less validity is found supporting any one of them.

Research on item difficulty/discrimination and standards for mastery has begun in CBM systems. However, the data should be viewed more as exemplary than definitive. The difficulty/ discrimination of items may be a function of the sampling procedures.

In using a CBM approach, the curriculum must be neither too easy, where the performance quickly would reach a ceiling, nor too difficult, where performance remains low, representing a floor effect. As in norm-referenced testing, the major issue in sampling items is the degree to which the test is likely to reflect performance changes.

As in traditional criterion-referenced testing, goal mastery in CBM approaches has been premised more on logical than empirical grounds. Mirkin et al. (1981) suggested the following levels of performance standards in establishing a long-range goal level and in writing IEPs in reading: for students in grades 1 and 2, the student should read at a rate of 50 words per minute with two or fewer errors. For students in grades 3 through 6, the reading rates should be at least 100 words per minute with four errors or fewer.

The data supporting this standard are premised primarily on the informal but logical assertion noted above. A long-range goal for mastery should not be too easy or it will be mastered quickly and will need to be changed during the year (comparisons of performance before and after this change will be confounded with the measurement change, precluding any statements about instructional effects). But if the level of performance on long-range goal material is too low, no effects will be forthcoming, since the scale is not sensitive to low levels of change or improvement.

Item Domain Determination

Three studies have been completed that bear on the establishment of an appropriate domain. Tindal and Deno (1981) investigated the differential sensitivity of three-item generation methods in spelling. Specifically, they included one domain where words were sampled specific to the content of instruction, one that sampled words from the grade level of instruction, and a third that sampled words from across several grade levels. They found that the most sensitive domain (generating the steepest slope) came from the domain that focused on instruction. However, this domain also generated considerable variability. The domain that sampled items from within the grade level of instruction, although exhibiting a less noticeable slope of change, also resulted in less variability, making it very relevant for generating IEP objectives.

Similar results were found in a study by Fuchs, Tindal, and Deno (1981). More sensitive measures were generated from domains that reflected the content of instruction. Again, increased variability was present. Further, Fuchs et al. found that sample duration also influenced student performance: longer measures generated more stable performance.

Fuchs and Fuchs (1986) compared the effects of two types of sampling plans: long-range or short-term goals. The former was defined as material in which proficiency was expected within the following 15 or more weeks. Short-term goals were defined as material that had been sequenced into small and hierarchically arranged segments, which the student was expected to master successively. Fuchs and Fuchs found no effect size associated with goal sampling (long or short term), but did find an interaction between them and the type of measures: within short-term measurement, the mean effect size for probe-like measures was 0.40 higher than that of global measures. Yet, for long-term goal measurement, the average effect size for probe-like measures was 0.51 lower than that of global measures. In essence, the domain for sampling items on an IEP is related to the format for measurement and the eventual gain produced.

Establishing Levels of Mastery

In the only study on goal mastery with a CBM criterion-referenced approach, Fuchs, Fuchs, and Deno (1985) analyzed teachers' long-range goals. Some of the goals later were categorized as "ambitious," and some were categorized as "not ambitious." They focused on the relationship between goal ambitiousness and the amount of gain subsequently found on posttest achievement. They found that teachers who established higher IEP goals also accomplished higher levels of achievement on the posttests. Since one of the criterion measures was an oral reading fluency measure, greater improvement may have been expected because it was so similar to the measurement condition of weekly oral reading on a passage. However, Fuchs et al. also found improvement on a published norm-referenced test, which was not biased in favor of an oral fluency format.

Empirical Results on Student Achievement with CRA

Fuchs, Deno, and Mirkin (1984) performed a study with 39 teachers in New York in which three outcome measures of reading achievement were collected. Half of the teachers were trained to write CBM long-range goals for their students, and half were allowed to monitor IEP goals as they wished. They found that "children whose teachers employed the ongoing measurement and evaluation system, DBPM, achieved better than students whose teachers used conventional monitoring methods" (p. 456).

Tindal and Shinn (1988) discovered that IEP goal mastery was related to improvement on CBM measures of reading and spelling administered three times during the year. In their study, special education students with complete CBM periodic and annual review data for all three testing periods (fall, winter, spring) were included, resulting in 60 students with IEPs in spelling and 86 students with IEPs in reading. The analysis compared improvement in their raw score performance on the assessment data collected in the fall and spring (gain scores) and their eventual mastery of the long-range goal stated in the IEPs. The question was whether students who mastered their IEP long-range goals also improved on a broader and more global measure, a norm-referenced CBM. Special education students who eventually mastered their IEP goals in reading and spelling achieved significantly higher performance levels relative to their peers on the CBM measures. A point biserial correlation, however, indicated that although this relationship was statistically significant, it was somewhat low in its magnitude of effect (0.20–0.30). As a proxy for achievement in general, mastery of specific IEP goals is related to overall growth in general: students who master their IEP goal improve more than other students who do not master their objective. Thus, CRA-type evaluation using mastery of objectives may be a promising approach to evaluation of programs.

Issues in Use of CRAs

Given the limited empirical basis for establishing a CRA and the preliminary outcome data on its use, some cautions are needed. Specifically, four issues should be considered in using this approach to evaluate special education programs: (1) definition of a domain that can reflect change and has potential for being mastered, (2) consideration of error rates in making decisions about mastery, (3) definition of the group to include in the evaluation, and (4) organization and analysis of data. As in the norm-referenced approach, these issues are interdependent.

Sensitivity to Change

In a CRA approach to program evaluation, domains must be written carefully to be sensitive to instructional outcomes. Since no standards are likely to be present (e.g., number of students in another program who master similar objectives), it is difficult to assay the appropriateness of the domain with certainty. As a consequence, interpretation of a program's effect is difficult. Ultimately, improvement on a criterion measure (the norm-referenced measures) may be employed, as in the research described earlier by Tindal and Shinn (1988). Alternatively, tracking individual students from one year to the next may be appropriate. However, since mastery ultimately is a judgmental process in either the selection of the domain and/or the standards or cutoff scores, this form of evaluation will always be suspect and in need of clarification (Glass, 1980).

Mastery Decision Errors

Another important issue in the use of a CRA is the lack of meaning to "mastery" without reference to the specific domain. As in all forms of criterion-referenced testing, the definition of mastery is elusive, with multiple interpretations. As Livingston and Zieky (1982) reported, many strategies can be used to establish passing or mastery scores. However, little is known about the reliability of most of these procedures.

Two types of errors, false positives and false negatives, are possible in making mastery decisions. False positives occur when the conclusion is made that a student has mastered the objective when, in fact, he/she has not mastered it. False negatives occur when the student is classified as not having mastered the objective when really he/she has mastered the objective. Fuchs, Fuchs, and Warren (1982) determined that teachers more often make the error that students have mastered material when in fact they have not. In a more task-analytic system, where a scope and sequence chart is used to progress the student through the curriculum, these errors may have bearing on the eventual learning of the skill sequence. There is the potential for development of splinter skills with false positives and loss of student progress with false negatives.

An additional concern about the mastery decision is the stability of the mastery scores. Little empirical data exist specifying how many days students must perform at the criterion level of the IEP goal before they can be considered as having mastered the material with a high degree of certainty. One must question the definition of mastery: Is one data point at the expected level sufficient to be considered as mastery, or are more data points at the expected levels needed?

Defining the Reference Group

Although the number of special education students who meet their IEP goals appears promising as a measure of program effectiveness, this group should be described clearly with a written rationale. In the data cited from Pine County, only students who had received special education services for the entire academic year were included. Students with IEPs developed after December 1 (the deadline for reporting children on the child count to the Federal government) were not included in the goal mastery summary. Although this strategy limited the report to only a subset of the number of children that teachers actually served, the results were more interpretable by their inclusion of only students served for a full year.

Data Organization and Analysis

In data reported for the 1982–83 academic year in Pine County, all special education teachers completed a computerized survey at the end of the year, noting the academic areas in which their students were served and the outcome of the instructional program relative to the IEP objective: whether the student mastered the goal. This form was used as the cover page for the data sheet for all individual CBM testing (i.e., eligibility testing, periodic and annual reviews). Although individual graphs of progress towards IEP objectives had been completed on each student, these data were not collected.

The number of students who met their IEP goals was calculated from the data-coding sheets. These results are summarized in Figure 8.4. In this particular evaluation, the number of students who mastered their goal exceeded the number who failed to meet their goals. These data also were summarized for each teacher and each school district within the special education cooperative (G. Germann, unpublished data).

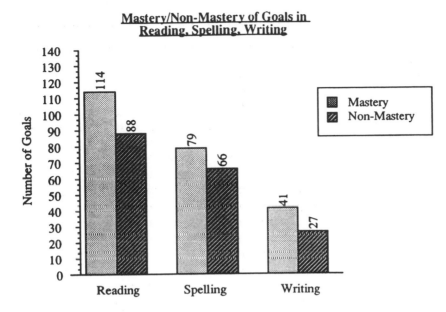

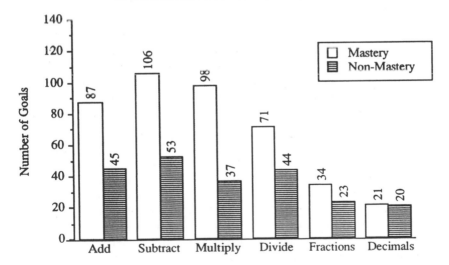

FIGURE 8.4. Number of goals from individual educational plans in four basic skill areas mastered and not mastered at the time of annual review.

Prescriptions and Conclusions on a CRA Evaluation

Because a criterion-referenced evaluation strategy relies on monitoring students' progress toward individual IEP goals, attention should be given to the quality of these goals and the fidelity of the student progress monitoring. A number of procedures can be used to define this level, including the criteria proposed by Mirkin et al. (1981), normative levels, or teacher judgment. As mentioned earlier, establishment of appropriate goals assumes that the measurement material is more encompassing than an immediate instructional level but not so distant that little overlap exists between instruction and measurement. Once teachers have begun to measure student performance on long-range goals, the only remaining issues are maintenance of the measurement procedures for the remainder of the year and the collection of objective mastery data at year's end, at which time teachers simply note whether or not the goal has been reached. The final two decisions that are considered are the composition of the student group (e.g., served all year or type of student) for whom to aggregate data and the level of aggregation (i.e., by IEP area, by teacher, building, district, etc.).

INDIVIDUAL-REFERENCED ASSESSMENTS

In the individual-referenced approach, changes in performance over time are summarized with each student. These changes are not compared to other students as in the norm-referenced approach, nor are they compared to an established or expected goal or standard, as in the criterion-referenced approach. Rather, performance is compared over time to previously attained performance levels.

Similar to a criterion-referenced assessment, the IRA approach is successful when it has a reliable, valid, and continuous system of monitoring progress. The CBM procedures described in Chapter 6 meet these criteria. Rather than using a single statement about mastery or nonmastery of the objective to summarize a program's final outcome, a number of dimensions of time-series data are summarized. All of the following are premised on repeated measurement over time: (1) slope of improvement, (2) variability in performance, (3) changes in median levels, (4) jump or step change, and (5) overlap. See Parsonson and Baer (1978) and

Tawney and Gast (1984) for a more complete description of indices.

Two systems have been proposed for measuring student performance repeatedly (Fuchs, 1986, 1987): (1) *progress-monitoring systems* require IEP measurement material to be sampled from successive instructional levels, and (2) *performance-monitoring systems* use material from long-range goal material. Individual-referenced approaches to program evaluation generally are more applicable for the latter strategy, in which performance consistently is monitored from a constant domain, not from a series of successive domains.

Summary Metrics and Their Applications

Slope of improvement, variability, and overlap are probably the most important dimensions to evaluate when data are collected over time. Slope indicates the general change in trend of student achievement, reflecting positive, negative, or no growth. Variability represents the consistency of student performance over time. High variability means that performance is erratic, whereas low variability indicates stable performance. Overlap refers to the band that encompasses common data values across successive phases and reflects the lack of change when it is high (Parsonson & Baer, 1978). This may represent the most comprehensive index in that it is a function of both slope and variability as well as any immediate changes in step.

Developing Aggregate Indices

This range of summary techniques, although increasing the flexibility for evaluating outcomes, also reduces the reliability of determining consistent outcomes (Tindal, 1982). Considerable disagreement often exists in making judgments about the effects of interventions between individuals and with those same individuals over two time periods. In part, this outcome may be a function of contradictions among the different indices. For example, a positive change in slope, indicating an improved trend in performance over time, also may be accompanied by an increase in variability, indicating less systematic performance from one measurement to the next. Unreliability also may result from the use of visual inspection for determining significant outcomes (Wampold & Furlong, 1981). With no firm guidelines and anchors for judging how much change is needed to constitute a "real" change, it is difficult for two people to agree on improvement.

A proposal and critique for summarizing single-subject research appears in a recent issue of *Remedial and Special Education*. As Scruggs, Mastropieri, and Castro (1987) noted, the most sensitive and meaningful datum for aggregating time-series performance across individuals is the amount (proportion) of nonoverlapping data between successive phases, particularly base line and treatment. They noted that in most single-subject research studies, the average number of data points within any treatment phase is fairly low, ranging from three to 10 data points, which would lend itself to this summary technique.

Basically, calculation of nonoverlap requires counting the number of data points in the treatment phase that fall above the highest data value occurring during previous phases or base-line phases. This number is subsequently divided by the total number of data points occurring during the treatment phase to convert it to a percentage metric. Scruggs et al. (1987) supported the overlap metric by stating that (1) it reflects slope, change in step, and variability at the same time; (2) it can be consistently applied across many different studies; and (3) it is quite robust to the many diverse issues in measurement (number of different data points, scales for displaying the data, and manner of calculation).

Although applicable in most single subject studies, this technique is difficult to execute. Scruggs et al. (1987) cited four specific instances: (1) when changes in slope in base-line and treatment phases are in the opposite direction, (2) when the base-line data reflect a trend in the direction expected only during the intervention, (3) when a "floor" or "ceiling" effect is attained, with all data points at a minimum or maximum level, respectively, and (4) in cases depicting very complex data arrays that limit the utility of summarizing the information in a single metric. Although this technique has been criticized (White, 1987; Salzberg, Strain, & Baer, 1987), Scruggs et al. defended its use as generally appropriate when data during the base-line and treatment phases include relatively few values, which they note is typical in much of the published literature appearing in the *Journal of Applied Behavior Analysis* from 1968 to 1977.

In lieu of evaluating programs with this datum, the most sensible procedure is to focus on slope of improvement, since it is the ultimate datum for viewing change in performance over time.

Little empirical data exist to help in the selection of either type of metric. The logical decision is to apply overlap if few data points are available or if considerable data are missing and to use average slope of performance if the data array is extensive and complete.

Aggregating Data

Time-series data from students' IEPs or their performance graphs are difficult to aggregate for two reasons. First, data files typically become so massive that many microcomputers are too small to handle the data. A second, related problem is the lack of software to aggregate the indices noted above: overlap, slope, or variability. These indices are not available on most software. Measures of overlap and variability of single-student performance also rarely are included as options in most software programs.

One solution is the Progress Monitoring Program (Germann, 1987). This software, compatible with an Apple II computer, summarizes the slope of improvement and variability for successive programs implemented within a student's IEP. Analyses can be based on either a "treatment-oriented" or "goal-oriented" analysis (Fuchs, 1987). In treatment-oriented analysis, the slopes of successive programs can be compared with each other. A goal-oriented analysis allows the slope of improvement to be compared to the goal established by the teacher at the outset of the program, with a percentage of goal attainment aim used to judge a program's effectiveness. Also, a teacher can aggregate the slopes directly across any group of individuals by age/grade, type of IEP, classification, etc.

Issues in the Use of an Individual-Referenced Assessment

Two issues appear in the use of an individual-referenced approach for evaluating educational programs: (1) identification of summarizing statistics that are appropriate and that provide valid interpretations and (2) establishment of procedures for reporting and interpreting data.

Summarizing Statistics

As reflected in the field of educational research, there has been considerable debate on summarizing time-series data. True time-series analyses appear to be inappropriate for use in the classroom, given the need for a large number of data points and complicated computational techniques (Box & Jenkins, 1976; McCain & McCleary, 1979). Although some argue for the use of parametric statistics to determine effects (Edgington, 1982; Gentile, Roden, & Klein, 1974; Huitema, 1985), others caution against their use, given the serial nature of the data (Kazdin, 1976).

Another major issue is the number of data points needed to determine a stable slope. As White (1971) noted, the accuracy of slope in predicting performance is, in part, a function of the number of data points used to summarize it. He suggested that 11 data points will generate an accurate prediction of performance in the short term (up to 2 weeks). In a recent study completed by Stein (1987), quarter-intersect slopes based on 24 data points collected over 8 weeks were quite accurate in predicting performance at the 12th week.

Establishing an Appropriate Comparison Standard

More fundamental problems than the psychometric issues involved in summarizing time-series data may be (1) the lack of an appropriate standard for determining whether special education programs are effective and (2) the use of a weak design for determining such effectiveness. Unless a pre-special-education standard can be generated, it is quite difficult to assay or interpret program outcomes. For any student, it may be that although performance does not improve much in special education, it is drastically better than it would have been without special education. Of course, this is very speculative, and arguments can be developed in support of or in contradistinction to such a contention. Therefore, more prereferral data must be generated in relation to outcomes from regular education to make this summary procedure sensible. However, even with this strategy, threats potentially invalidate any outcomes. Two very immediate and powerful issues relate to the fact that an order effect is present, in that prereferral interventions always appear first, and the fact that time, maturation, and multiple interventions are possible confounds (Cook & Campbell, 1979). Since the purpose in program evaluation, however, is less to determine cause than to mark outcomes, such concerns may be diminished in importance.

Empirical Results on Student Achievement

Only one study has been completed using a CBM individual-referenced approach in the evaluation of programs at the systems level. In a study completed by Brown, Magnusson, and Marston (1986) and published by Marston (1987–1988), fourth-, fifth-, and sixth-grade students initially were identified as in regular education but "at risk," below the 15th percentile on a series of locally developed criterion-referenced tests. From this group of students, approximately 25 were selected as having a high probability of being placed in special education with reading problems; they were tested systematically in reading over 6 weeks, and the slope of improvement was calculated. Eventually, 11 students from this group were actually placed in special education and had IEPs developed in reading; again, the slope of improvement was determined over a 6-week period. In a basic AB design, with A representing regular education and B representing special education, an evaluation was conducted on the differences between the 6-week slopes in the two settings. In regular education, the average slope of improvement was 0.60 word increase per week, whereas 6 weeks of weekly data denerated a slope of 1.15 word increase per week in special education. Using a repeated-measures analysis of varience, they found significant differences in the average slopes across these two environments.

Summary and Prescriptions

The use of individual-referenced approaches to evaluating educational programs has been confined to the individual student level, rarely appearing in overall systems-level evaluations. Yet, as demonstrated in the study by Marston (1987–88), this approach is sensible and should be more readily considered. Obviously, it requires more systematic data collection and monitoring, thereby making it more prone to being ignored or, worse, being completed incorrectly or inaccurately.

Prescriptions for an IRA Evaluation

The first step in the use of such a procedure is to ensure that as much complete data be generated as possible, with minimal missing data. A collection procedure then must be developed for obtaining data from all teachers. The only manageable system to appear to date employs a microcomputer program with an Apple II (PMP; Germann, 1987). These data then are aggregated systematically to generate an overall slope. The use of two phases, one in regular education and the other in special education, appears to be an excellent idea that has yet to be implemented. Therefore, the only summary report typical from this approach is the average slope. This datum, however, means very little without reference to either some description of the sampling domains employed in the generation of the slope or an anchor for interpreting it: the slope from previous years or the slope generated in regular education. Clearly, the former anchor is more in keeping with the premise of this approach, using the student as his/her own comparison and relating improvement over time to previous levels.

SUMMARY

The purpose of this chapter was to review procedures for evaluating educational programs, with an emphasis on using three different assessment approaches: norm-, criterion-, and individual-referenced. The important difference among these three strategies was defined as the manner in which data are interpreted. In a norm-referenced approach, two groups of students are compared, typically regular and special education. In a criterion-referenced approach, the anchor for making comparisons is a benchmark or standard for mastery which can be derived in a variety of ways. Finally, in an individual-referenced approach, student performance is compared to itself over time.

Each strategy is premised on different data, typically collected in a different manner from each other. Clearly, the norm-referenced approach employs the broadest domain and the least frequent schedule of measurement. In most districts employing this technique, data are collected on grade-level tasks three times per year. In both the criterion-referenced and individual-referenced approaches, data are collected from long-range goal measurement material deemed appropriate for the student's IEP; frequency of measurement is far more regular, often completed at least weekly. At the systems level, however, summaries are inherently summative and are completed at the end of the year in all three strategies.

A number of issues have been considered throughout the chapter in each of the three approaches—reviewing the underlying considerations including logistic and psychometric problems, summarizing the available empirical data, and providing prescriptions on their application in the public schools. In the end, any program evaluation should incorporate all three approaches to avoid the limitations of any one of them.

ACKNOWLEDGMENT

Richard Parker and Jan Hasbrouck, doctoral students from the University of Oregon, formatted the graphs in Figure 8.3.

REFERENCES

Angoff, W. H. (1971). Scales, norms, and equivalent scores. In R. L. Thorndike (Ed.), *Educational measurement* (pp. 514–515). Washington: American Council on Education.

Borich, G., & Nance, D. D. (1987). Evaluating special education programs: Shifting the professional mandate from process to outcome. *Remedial and Special Education, 8,* 7–16.

Box, G. E. P., & Jenkins, G. M. (1976). *Time series analysis: Forecasting and control.* San Francisco: Holden Day.

Brown, J., Magnusson, D., & Marston, D. (1986). *The effectiveness of special education: A time series analysis of performance in regular and special education settings.* Unpublished manuscript, Minneapolis Public Schools, 254 Upton Avenue South, Minneapolis, MN 55405.

Brzeinski, J., & Schoephoerster, H. (1981). *Towers: Test of basic reading skills.* Boston: Houghton-Mifflin.

Cook, T. D., & Campbell, D. T. (1979). *Quasi-experimentation: Design and analysis issues for field settings.* Chicago: Rand McNally.

Deno, S. L., & Mirkin, P. K. (1977). *Data-based program modification: A manual.* Reston, VA: Council for Exceptional Children.

Deno, S. L., Mirkin, P. K., Chiang B., & Lowry, L. (1980). *Relationships among simple measures of reading and performance on standardized achievement tests* (Research Report No. 20). Minneapolis: University of Minnesota Institute for Research on Learning Disabilities.

Deno, S. L., Mirkin, P. K., Lowry, L., & Kuehnle, K. (1980). *Relationships among simple measures of reading and performance on standardized achievement tests* (Research Report No. 21). Minneapolis: University of Minnesota Institute for Research on Learning Disabilities.

Deno, S. L., Mirkin, P. K., & Marston, D. (1980). *Relationships among simple measures of written expression and performance on standardized achievement tests* (Research Report No. 22). Minneapolis: University of Minnesota Institute for Research on Learning Disabilities.

Durr, W. K., LePere, J. M., & Pikulski, J. J. (1981). *Houghton Mifflin reading program: Towers.* Boxton: Houghton Mifflin.

Ebel, R. I. (1972). *Essentials of educational measurement.* Englewood Cliffs, NJ: Prentice-Hall.

Edgington, E. S. (1982). Nonparametric tests for single-subject multiple schedule experiments. *Behavioral Assessment, 4,* 83–91.

Fitz-Gibbons, C. T., & Morris, L. L. (1978). *How to design a program evaluation.* Beverly Hills, CA: Sage Publications.

Fuchs, D., & Fuchs, L. S. (1986). Effects of systematic formative evaluation: A metaanalysis. *Exceptional Children, 53,* 199–208.

Fuchs, D., Fuchs, L. S., Benowitz, S., & Berringer, K. (1987). Norm-referenced tests: Are they valid for use with handicapped students? *Exceptional Children, 54,* 263–271.

Fuchs, L. S. (1986). Monitoring progress among mildly handicapped pupils: Review of current practice and research. *Remedial and Special Education, 7,* 5–12.

Fuchs, L. S. (1987). Program development. *Teaching Exceptional Children, 20*(1), 42–44.

Fuchs, L., Deno, S. L., & Mirkin, P. K. (1984). The effects of frequent curriculum-based measurement and evaluation on pedagogy, student achievement, and student awareness of learning. *American Educational Research Journal, 21,* 449–460.

Fuchs, L. S., Fuchs, D., & Deno, S. (1985). The importance of goal ambitiousness and goal mastery to student achievement. *Exceptional Children, 52,* 63–71.

Fuchs, L., Fuchs, D., & Warren, L. M. (1982). *Special education practice in evaluating student progress toward goals* (Research Report No. 82). Minneapolis: University of Minnesota Institute for Research on Learning Disabilities (ERIC Document Reproduction Service No. ED 224 198).

Fuchs, L. S., Tindal, G., & Deno, S. (1981). *Effects of varying item domain and sample duration on technical characteristics of daily measure in reading* (Research Report No. 48). Minneapolis: University of Minnesota Institute for Research on Learning Disabilities.

Gentile, J. R., Roden, A. H., & Klein, R. D. (1974). An analysis of variance model for the intrasubject replication design. *Journal of Applied Behavior Analysis, 5,* 193–198.

Germann, G. (1987). *Progress Monitoring Program* [computer program]. Sandstone, MN: Pine County Special Education Cooperative.

Gersten, R., & Hauser, C. (1984). The case for impact evaluations in special education. *Remedial and Special Education 5,* 16–24.

Glass, G. (1978). Standards and criteria. *Journal of Educational Measurement, 15,* 237–261.

Glass, G. (1980). When educators set standards. In E. L. Baker & E. S. Quellmalz (Eds.), *Educational testing and evaluation* (pp. 185–193). Beverly Hills, CA: Sage Publications.

Horst, D. P., Tallmadge, G. K., & Wood, C. T. (1975). *A practical guide to measuring project impact on student achievement* (Monograph No. 1 on evaluation in education). Washington: U.S. Government Printing Office.

Huitema, B. E. (1985). Autocorrelation in applied behavior analysis: A myth. *Behavioral Assessment, 7,* 109–120.

Kazdin, A. E. (1976). Statistical analysis of single-case experimental designs.

In M. Hersen & D. Barlow (Eds.), *Single case experimental designs: Strategies for studying behavior change* (pp. 265–316). New York: Pergamon Press.

Livingston, S. A. (1980). Choosing minimum passing scores by stochastic approximation techniques. *Educational and Psychological Measurement, 40,* 859–873.

Livingston, S. A., & Zieky, M. J. (1982). *Passing scores: A manual for setting standards of performance on educational and occupational tests.* Princeton, NJ: Educational Testing Service.

Maher, C. A., & Barbrack, C. R. (1979). Perspectives and principles for the evaluation of special-service programs. *The Journal of Special Education, 13,* 413–420.

Marston, D. (1987–1988). The effectiveness of special education: A time series analysis of reading performance in regular and special education. *The Journal of Special Education, 21,* 13–26.

McCain, M. J., & McCleary, R. (1979). The statistical analysis of the simple interrupted time series quasi-experiment. In T. D. Cook & D. T. Campbell (Eds.), *Quasiexperimentation: Design and analysis issues for field settings.* (pp. 233–294). Chicago: Rand McNally.

Mirkin, P. K., Deno, S. L., Fuchs, L. S., Wesson, C., Tindal, G., Marston, D., & Kuehnle, K. (1981). *Procedures to develop and monitor progress on IEP goals.* Minneapolis: University of Minnesota Institute for Research on Learning Disabilities.

Nedelsky, L. (1954). Absolute grading standards for objective tests. *Educational and Psychological Measurement, 14,* 3–19.

Parsonson, B. S., & Baer, D. M. (1978). The analysis and presentation of graphic data. In T. R. Kratochwill (Ed.), *Single subject research: Strategies for evaluating change* (pp. 101–166). New York: Academic Press.

Popham, W. J. (1978). *Criterion-referenced measurement.* Englewood Cliffs, NJ: Prentice Hall.

Salzberg, C., Strain, P., & Baer, D. (1987). Meta-analysis for single-subject research: When does it clarify, when does it obscure? *Remedial and Special Education, 8,* 43–48.

Scruggs, T., Mastropieri, M., & Castro, G. (1987). The quantitative synthesis of single-subject research: Methodology and validation. *Remedial and Special Education, 8,* 24–33.

Shinn, M. R. (1986). Does anyone really care what happens after the refer–test–place sequence: The systematic evaluation of special education program effectiveness. *School Psychology Review, 15,* 49–58.

Stake, R. (1976). The countenance of educational evaluation. *Teachers College Record, 68,* 523–540.

Stein, S. (1987). *Accuracy in predicting student reading performance based on time series progress monitoring data.* Unpublished doctoral dissertation, University of Oregon, Eugene, OR.

Stufflebeam, D. L., Foley, R., Gephart, W. J., Guba, E. G., Hammond, H. D., Merriman, H. O., & Provus, M. M. (1971). *Educational evaluation and decision making.* Itasca, IL: Peacock.

Tallmadge, G. K. (1981). An empirical assessment of norm-referenced evaluation methodology. *Journal of Educational Measurement, 19,* 97–112.

Tawney, J. W., & Gast, D. L. (1984). *Single subject research in special education.* Columbus, OH: Charles E. Merrill.

Tindal, G. (1982). *Visual analysis of time series data.* Unpublished doctoral dissertation, University of Minnesota, Minneapolis.

Tindal, G., & Deno, S. L. (1981). *Daily measurement of reading: Effects of varying the size of the item pool* (Research Report No. 55). Minneapolis: University of Minnesota Institute for Research on Learning Disabilities.

Tindal, G., Germann, G., & Deno, S. L. (1983). *Descriptive research on the Pine County norms: A compilation of findings.* Minneapolis: University of Minnesota Institute for Research on Learning Disabilities.

Tindal, G., Germann, G., Marston, D., & Deno, S. L. (1983). *The effectiveness of special education: A direct measurement approach.* (Research Report No. 123). Minneapolis: University of Minnesota Institute for Research on Learning Disabilities.

Tindal, G., & Shinn, M. R. (1983). [Relationship between mastery of long range goals and improvement on normative measures]. Unpublished raw data.

Tindal, G., Shinn, M. R., & Germann, G. (1987). The effect of different metrics on interpretation of change in program evaluation. *Remedial and Special Education, 8,* 14–28.

Wampold, B., & Furlong, M. (1981). The heuristics of visual inference. *Behavioral Assessment, 3,* 79–92.

White, O. (1971). *A pragmatic approach to the description of progress in the single case.* Unpublished doctoral dissertation, University of Oregon, Eugene.

White, O. (1987). Some comments concerning "The quantitative synthesis of single subject research." *Remedial and Special Education, 8,* 34–39.

APPENDIX
Administration and Scoring Procedures for Reading, Written Expression, Spelling, and Mathematics

SPECIFIC DIRECTIONS FOR READING

Setting of Data Collection

The reading measures must be administered to students individually. Prepare two copies of each passage, a numbered copy for examiner use and an unnumbered copy for the student to read.

Directions

Say to the student: *"When I say 'start,' begin reading aloud at the top of this page. Read across the page* [demonstrate by pointing]. *Try to read each word. If you come to a word you don't know, I'll tell it to you. Be sure to do your best reading. Are there any questions?"*

Say *"Start."*

Follow along on your copy of the story, marking the words that are read incorrectly. If a student stops or struggles with a word for 3 seconds, tell the student the word and mark it as incorrect.

Place a vertical line after the last word read and thank the student.

Count the number of words read correctly and incorrectly.

Scoring

The most important piece of information is the number of words read correctly. Reading fluency is a combination of speed and accuracy.

1. *Words read correctly.* Words read correctly are those words that are pronounced correctly, given the reading context.
   a. The word "read" must be pronounced "reed" when presented in the context of "He will read the book," not as "red."
   b. Repetitions are not counted as incorrects.

    c. Self-corrections within 3 seconds are counted as correctly read words.
2. *Words read incorrectly.* The following types of errors are counted: (a) mispronunciations, (b) substitutions, and (c) omissions. Further, words not read within 3 seconds are counted as errors.
    a. *Mispronunciations* are words that are misread: *dog* for *dig.*
    b. *Substitutions* are words that are substituted for the stimulus word; this is often inferred by a one-to-one correspondence between word orders: *dog* for *cat.*
    c. *Omissions* are words skipped or not read; if a student skips an entire line, each word is counted as an error.
3. *3-Second rule.* If a student is struggling to pronounce a word or hesitates for 3 seconds, the student is told the word, and it is counted as an error.

SPECIFIC DIRECTIONS FOR WRITTEN EXPRESSION

Setting of Data Collection

The written expression measures can be administered to students individually or in groups. Have a copy of the story starter or topic sentence available.

Directions

Say to the student: *"I want you to write a story. I am going to read a sentence to you first, and then I want you to write a short story about what happens. You will have 1 minute to think about the story you will write and then have 3 minutes to write it. Do your best work. If you don't know how to spell a word, you should guess. Are there any questions?"*

    "For the next minute, think about . . . [insert the story starter].*"*

    After 1 minute is up, say *"Start writing."*

    After 3 minutes, say *"Stop and put your pencil down."*

Scoring

Currently, there are four options for scoring.

1. *Total words written.* Count the total number of words written during the 3-minute period, including the words that are spelled incorrectly. Do not count numbers that are not spelled out (1987, 3, 29) as words. Be sure to count the title if written and proper names and nouns as words. If the student writes the story starter as part of the story, be sure to include those words in the count.
2. *Words spelled correctly.* Count the number of words spelled correctly. A word is counted as spelled correctly if it can stand alone as a word in the English language. Do not spend a lot of time trying to infer what specific word the student "meant." If it is a recognizable word and it is spelled correctly, count it.

3. *Total letters written.* Use the same criterion as counting total words except count the number of letters written, whether the words are spelled correctly or not. Do not count numbers.
4. *Correct word sequences.* This procedure takes more time than the other three. If "word salads" are generated, this method can provide a useful index of meaningful content. Count as a word sequence the joining of two words together that are spelled correctly and are grammatically correct. Do not count numbers next to words in the total.

SPECIFIC DIRECTIONS FOR SPELLING

Setting of Data Collection

The spelling measures may be administered to students individually or in groups. Have the words to be dictated selected in advance. Use 10-second intervals for younger students (grades 1–3). Use a 7-second interval between words for older students (grades 4–8).

Directions

Say to the student: *"I am going to read some words to you. I want you to write the words on the sheet in front of you. Write the first word on the first line, the second word on the second line, and so on. I'll give you 10 seconds to spell each word. When I say the next word, try to write it, even if you haven't finished the last one. Are there any questions?"*
    Say the first word and start timing.
    Say each word twice. Use homonyms in a sentence.
    Say a new word every 10 (or 7) seconds.
    Dictate words for 2 minutes. About 12–13 words should be presented if words are dictated every 10 seconds. About 17–18 words should be presented if words are dictated every 7 seconds. Do not dictate a new word in the last 3 seconds and allow the student to finish the last word.

SPECIFIC DIRECTIONS FOR MATH

Setting of Data Collection

The math measures can be administered to students individually or in groups. Note whether single-skill or multiple-skill probes are to be administered.

Directions

Say to the student: *"The sheets on your desk are math facts."*
    For single-skill probes say: *"All of the problems are* [addition or subtraction or multiplication or division] *facts."*
    For multiple-skill probes say: *"There are several types of problems on the sheet.*

Some are addition, some are subtraction, some are multiplication, and some are division [as appropriate]. *Look at each problem carefully before you answer it."*

"When I say 'start,' Turn them over and begin answering the problems. Start on the first problem on the left on the top row [point]. Work across and then go to the next row. If you can't answer the problem make an 'X' on it and to to the next one. If you finish one side, go to the back. Are there any questions?"

Say *"Start."*

Monitor student performance so that students work the problems in rows and do not skip around or answer only the easy problems.

After 2 minutes, say *"Stop."*

Scoring

Count the number of correctly written digits in the problems. Place value is important. In the more complicated problems, one has to assign "point values" based on the longest method a student can be taught to use to solve a problem.

Index